A. Pouplard-Barthelaix   J. Emile
Y. Christen (Eds.)

Immunology
and Alzheimer's Disease

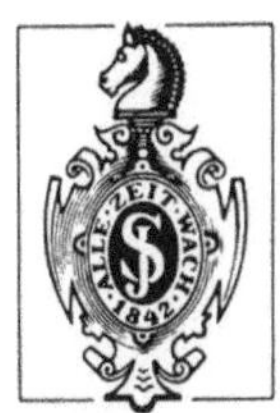

Springer-Verlag
Berlin Heidelberg New York
London Paris Tokyo

Pouplard-Barthelaix, Annick, Dr.
Unité de Neuro-Immunologie
et Neuropathologie et INSERM U. 298,
C.H.R.U, 49033 Angers Cedex,
France

Emile, Jean, Pr.
Service de Neurologie
C.H.R.U., 49033 Angers Cedex,
France

Christen, Yves, Dr.
Fondation IPSEN
pour la Recherche Thérapeutique,
30, rue Cambronne 75737 Paris Cedex,
France

ISBN-13: 978-3-642-46636-6   e-ISBN-13: 978-3-642-46634-2
DOI: 10.1007/978-3-642-46634-2

Preface

A great challenge of our time, Alzheimer's disease is one of the major concerns of the Fondation Ipsen pour la Recherche Thérapeutique. The Fondation Ipsen was created in 1983. Its essential purpose is to involve itself in areas of biomedicine where interdisciplinary collaboration is needed. Some of its objectives include putting leading physicians and scientists in touch with each other, publishing important works, and helping young researchers.

The Fondation Ipsen has already undertaken a large variety of initiatives, for example, by organizing several international colloquia on prostacyclin, atrial natriuretic Factor, PAF-acether, and cytoprotection (the series "Colloques Médecine et Recherche"). In the same spirit, it awards an annual prize and grant to specialists for the study of Alzheimer's disease. It also publishes documents on this disorder for the use of physicians and families involved.

With the international colloquium dedicated to the immunological aspects of Alzheimer's disease and cerebral amyloidosis organized at Angers on 14 September 1987, the Fondation Ipsen inaugurated a new round of activities: specialized meetings on the most up-to-date aspects of current research on Alzheimer's disease. The second in this series is the meeting on the genetic origins of Alzheimer's disease, scheduled for 25 March 1988 in Paris. Other events will follow, each with the objective of bringing together the most highly involved researchers and physicians in order to contribute to a real advance in knowledge.

Reports on the high-level scientific meetings will be published by Springer-Verlag in a new series of works, *Research and Perspectives in Alzheimer's Disease.*

Yves Christen
Vice-President of the Fondation Ipsen pour la Recherche Thérapeutique.

Acknowledgements. The editors wish to thanks Mrs Mary Gage for editorial assistance, Mrs Jacqueline Mervaillie for the organization of the meeting in Angers and Marie-Madeleine Portier, Philippe Brachet, Yvon Lamour and J. Urbain for their collaboration as chairmen of the meeting.

Contents

     Contents

Contributors

Barcikowska, M.
  Department of Neurology, Warsaw Medical Academy,
  Warsaw, Poland

Beer, J.
  Center for Molecular Biology, University of Heidelberg, 6900 Heidelberg, FRG

Beyreuther, K.
  Center for Molecular Biology, University of Heidelberg, 6900 Heidelberg, FRG

Cramer, M.
  Center for Molecular Biology, University of Heidelberg, 6900 Heidelberg, FRG

Currie, J. R.
  New York State Office of Mental Retardation and
  Developmental Disabilities, Institute for Basic Research in Developmental
  Disabilities, 1050 Forest Hill Road, Staten Island New York 10314, USA

Defossez, A.
  Laboratoire d'Histologie, Unité INSERM No. 156, Faculté de Médecine,
  59045 Lille Cedex, France

Delacourte, A.
  Laboratoire de Neurosciences, Unité INSERM No. 16, Faculté de Médecine,
  59045 Lille Cedex, France

Dyrks, T.
  Center for Molecular Biology, University of Heidelberg, 6900 Heidelberg, FRG

Eikelenboom, P.
  Department of Psychiatry, Medical Faculty, Free University, Amsterdam,
  The Netherlands

Fischer, P.
  Center for Molecular Biology, University of Heidelberg, 6900 Heidelberg, FRG

Fraser, H.
AFRC and MRC Neuropathogenesis Unit, West Mains Road, Edinburgh,
United Kingdom

Fudenberg, H. H.
Department of Microbiology and Immunology, Medical University
of South Carolina, 171 Ashley Avenue, Charleston, SC 29425, USA

Fuller, S.
Department of Pathology,
University of Western Australia and Department of Neuropathology,
Royal Perth Hospital, Perth, Australia

Genthe, A.
Center for Molecular Biology, University of Heidelberg, 6900 Heidelberg, FRG

Glenner, G. G.
Department of Pathology, University of California at San Diego,
School of Medicine, La Jolla, CA 92093, USA

Haga, S.
Psychiatric Research Institute of Tokyo,
Kamikitazawa 2–1–8, Setagaya-Ku, Tokyo, Japan 156

Hilbich, C.
Center for Molecular Biology, University of Heidelberg, 6900 Heidelberg, FRG

Horsthemke, B.
Institute of Humangenetic, University of Essen, Essen, FRG

Hutchinson, L.
Department of Pathology,
University of Western Australia and Department of Neuropathology,
Royal Perth Hospital, Perth, Australia

Ishii, T.
Psychiatric Research Institute of Tokyo, Kamikitazawa 2–1–8,
Setagaya-Ku, Tokyo, Japan 156

Kametani, F.
Psychiatric Research Institute of Tokyo,
Kamikitazawa 2–1–8, Setagaya-Ku, Tokyo, Japan 156

Martins, R.
Department of Pathology,
University of Western Australia and Department of Neuropathology,
Royal Perth Hospital, Perth, Australia

Masters, C. L.
Department of Pathology,
University of Western Australia and Department of Neuropathology,
Royal Perth Hospital, Perth, Australia

Miller, D. L.
New York State Office of Mental Retardation and
Developmental Disabilities,
Institute for Basic Research in Developmental Disabilities,
1050 Forest Hill Road, Staten Island, New York 10314, USA

Miyakawa, T.
Department of Neuropsychiatry, Kumamoto University Medical School,
Honjo Machi, Kumamoto, Japan

Monning, U.
Center for Molecular Biology, University of Heidelberg, 6900 Heidelberg, FRG

Multhaup, G.
Center for Molecular Biology, University of Heidelberg, 6900 Heidelberg, FRG

Pouplard-Barthelaix, A.
Unité de Neuro-Immunologie et Neuropathologie,
INSERM U. 298, C.H.R.U., 49033 Angers Cedex, France

Robakis, N. K.
New York State Office of Mental Retardation and
Developmental Disabilities,
Institute for Basic Research in Developmental Disabilities,
1050 Forest Hill Road, Staten Island, New York 10314, USA

Rozemuller, J. M.
Departments of Psychiatry and Neuropathology,
Medical Faculty, Free University, Amsterdam, The Netherlands

Rumble, B.
Department of Pathology,
University of Western Australia and Department of Neuropathology,
Royal Perth Hospital, Perth, Australia

Salbaum, J. M.
Center for Molecular Biology, University of Heidelberg, 6900 Heidelberg, FRG

Selkoe, D. J.
Department of Neurology (Neuroscience),
Harvard Medical School and Center for Neurological Diseases,
Brigham and Women's Hospital, Boston, MA 02115, USA

Simms, G.
Department of Pathology,
University of Western Australia and Department of Neuropathology,
Royal Perth Hospital, Perth, Australia

Singh, V. K.
Department of Microbiology and Immunology,
Medical University of South Carolina,
171 Ashley Avenue, Charleston, SC 29425, USA

Stam, F. C.
Department of Neuropathology, Medical Faculty, Free University,
Amsterdam, The Netherlands

Wehr, S.
Center for Molecular Biology, University of Heidelberg, 6900 Heidelberg, FRG

Weidemann, A.
Center for Molecular Biology, University of Heidelberg, 6900 Heidelberg, FRG

Wisniewski, H. M.
New York State Office of Mental Retardation and
Developmental Disabilities,
Institute for Basic Research in Developmental Disabilities,
1050 Forest Hill Road, Staten Island, New York 10314, USA

Zabel, P.
University of Mainz

Alzheimer's Disease, a Cerebral Form of Amyloidosis

H. M. Wisniewski, J. R. Currie, M. Barcikowska[1], N. K. Robakis, and *D. L. Miller*

Summary

Recent data suggest that amyloidosis of the brain is the cause of the cognitive pathology in Alzheimer's disease. The difference between normal aged individuals and those affected by Alzheimer's disease or senile dementia of Alzheimer's type (AD, SDAT) appears to be quantitative and topographic. Acceptance of the concept that AD and SDAT are a form of brain amyloidosis has both practical and theoretical consequences. The search for the amyloid-stimulating and -enhancing factors may lead to discovery of the cause of Alzheimer's disease. The development of treatment strategies must include a search for ways of inhibiting and/or activating the cells producing and/or processing aging-Alzheimer-amyloidogenic protein (AAAP) as well as methods which may help to remove the deposits of amyloid fibers.

For many years senile dementia, popularly called senility, was regarded as a natural, inevitable consequence of growing old. It is now believed that this is not the case. Instead, senile dementia is an age-associated disease. Today there are 25 million individuals in the United States who are aged 65 or older. Most estimates for the prevalence of the severer degrees of dementia among persons over 65 lie between 5% and 8%, and the lifetime cumulative risk of becoming severely demented by the age of 80 has been computed to lie between 15% and 20% (WHO 1986). It is estimated that about 50% of nursing home beds in the United States are now occupied by the severely demented. Because vital functions are generally spared, these severely demented people may survive for many years after the onset of the disease, and thus this disease extracts an enormous emotional and financial toll from relatives and friends.

There are many conditions that lead to senile dementia, however; the most common is senile dementia of the Alzheimer type (SDAT) (Wisniewski and Soifer 1979; Katzman 1981; Reisberg et al. 1985). Diagnosis of Alzheimer's disease (AD) is based on the presence of the clinical signs and symptoms of progressive dementia and the presence of many senile plaques containing amyloid and neurons filled with neurofibrillary tangles (composed, by and large, of paired helical filaments or PHF). Both the amyloid fibers and PHF show green birefringence when stained with Congo red. Both the PHF and amyloid deposits, when stained with thioflavine-S and examined by

---

[1] Dr. Barcikowska is a visiting scientist from the Warsaw Medical Academy, Department of Neurology, Warsaw, Poland

fluorescence microscopy, show characteristic yellow-green fluorescence. Plaque and vascular amyloid and PHF, like other amyloid fibers in systemic or localized amyloidosis, show beta-pleated sheet conformation (Glenner 1981; Selkoe 1987). The common characteristics of amyloid deposits are that they are aggregates of proteinaceous beta-pleated fibers and have common optical properties when stained with certain dyes. In spite of having similar optical properties, however, these fibers show great chemical diversity. The common optical properties of PHF and plaque amyloid, and their concomitant occurrence in aged and AD-affected brains were the source of several unitary theories (Divry 1934; von Braunmuhl 1957) concerning the pathogenesis of plaque formation and neurofibrillary changes. Recently, based on biochemical studies of the isolated cores of plaque amyloid, Beyreuther and Masters et al. (this volume) postulated that a common protein, the A-4 peptide, or β-protein, is the protein forming both the PHF and the plaque and vascular amyloid fibers.

Data from our institute, as well as from Drs. Glenner, Selkoe, and Delacourte's laboratories (this volume), do not support Beyreuther's and Masters' reports. The fine structure of PHF, as well as its protein biochemistry and immunochemistry, appear to be very different from the plaque and vascular amyloid fibers (Glenner and Wong 1986; Grundke-Iqbal et al. 1986a, b; Iqbal et al. 1987; Selkoe 1987; Wisniewski and Wrzolek 1987; Wisniewski et al. 1987a).

Neuritic (senile) plaques containing β-amyloid protein fibers are found only in old humans and animals, and in people with AD and Down's syndrome (DS). However, PHF of the type seen in AD are found only in certain neurons of the human brain. They occur in many etiologically unrelated diseases (Wisniewski and Soifer 1979), and their topographic distribution appears to be the same irrespective of the disease process. Therefore, PHF are region-specific rather than disease-specific. Recent studies using immunological and biochemical methods showed the following proteins to be present in the neurofibrillary tangles made of PHF: abnormally phosphorylated tau, ubiquitin, and neurofilaments (Sternberger et al. 1985; Grundke-Iqbal et al. 1986b; Mori et al. 1987; Selkoe 1987). However, difficulties in obtaining sufficient quantities of PHF for biochemical analysis have prevented the carrying out of proper quantitative studies to determine which of the PHF-associated protein(s) is the major protein component of the neurofibrillary tangles in AD. Recent studies by Terry et al. (1987) have shown that there is a large group (30%) of people over the age of 74 with SDAT who lack neocortical tangles. In our studies on the dynamics of plaque and tangle formation in individuals with DS, we found that the neuritic (senile) plaques occur much earlier in the brains of those affected with DS than do the neurofibrillary tangles (Wisniewski et al. 1987a, b, c). These results, and the fact that PHF may develop independently of plaques in other diseases, support in our opinion, the notion that the amyloid fiber protein and PHF protein(s) are different.

The recent rapid progress in the studies of the gene and protein forming the amyloid fibers in the vessels and plaques has been possible because of the report by Glenner and Wong (1984) of the purification and partial sequencing of the cerebrovascular amyloid peptide. Glenner and Wong called this novel protein, β-protein. In the literature this protein has also been called the Glenner peptide, or the A-4 protein (Wisniewski et al. 1986; Kang et al. 1987). Having the sequence of the β-protein, three laboratories working independently simultaneously reported the discovery of the cDNAs encoding the β-protein precursor (Goldgaber et al. 1987;

Kang et al. 1987; Robakis et al. 1987b). Sequencing of a full-length cDNA (Robakis et al. 1987a) has revealed that the β-protein precursor which we call aging-Alzheimer-amyloidogenic protein (AAAP) is a 695 amino acid polypeptide (Kang et al. 1987). In situ hybridization using a cDNA clone encoding the β-protein as a probe showed that in the central nervous system (CNS) the amyloid precursor mRNA is present in neurons, meninges, pericytes, endothelial cells, epithelial cells, and astrocytes. Outside the CNS, the mRNA was found in the kidneys, the heart, the lungs, and the liver.

Antibodies to synthetically made AAAP peptides (residues 98–116, 309–330, 420–430, 573–596, 649–671, 672–695) have demonstrated the presence of AAAP in many structures: adventitial and perivascular areas of meningeal and penetrating cortical vessels, pia-arachnoid, glia-limitans, reactive astroglia, large neurons, and the capsule and loose connective tissue in the spleen and the liver (Currie et al. 1987a). In addition, in the aged and AD-affected brain, anti-β-peptide polyclonal and monoclonal antibodies strongly labeled vascular amyloid deposits, the periphery (halo) of the classical plaques, and weakly, or not at all, the central core. Antisera to other AAAP peptides listed above do not label the classical plaques. Immunochemical differences between the isolated vascular amyloid peptide and the isolated core peptide have been revealed in ELISA studies using various antisera and monoclonal antibodies raised against the synthetic Glenner peptide sequences (Currie et al. 1987b). Biochemical studies of the core and vascular amyloid peptides have demonstrated some differences in solubility and amino acid residues between plaque core and vessel amyloids. The amino-terminus is blocked in the plaque core amyloid peptide, whereas in the cerebrovascular amyloid peptide it is not blocked; the plaque cores are insoluble in neutral guanidine HCl, while the vessel amyloid is soluble in neutral guanidine HCl (Bobin et al. 1987). From these data we have concluded that the differences between vascular and plaque core amyloid reflect either different routes of processing before the peptides are deposited or are the result of "aging" of the amyloid in the cores (Wisniewski and Miller 1986; Currie et al. 1987b). The role of the AAAP in normal brain function is unknown; however its presence among the connective tissue elements suggests that one of its functions may be as a junctional or extracellular matrix protein.

According to the current concepts based on studies of systemic amyloidosis, the formation of amyloid fibers is a two-step process involving the *production* of amyloidogenic protein, which is further *processed*, either locally or at distant sites, to yield amyloid fibers. This concept is supported by the observation that, in the majority of amyloidosis, one type of cell produces the amyloidogenic proteins, e. g., hepatocytes in secondary amyloidosis, or B cells in multiple myeloma, and that different cells (the reticuloendothelial cells) process the protein (Wegelius 1976; Glenner 1981; Wisniewski and Wrzolek 1987). From these data a unifying concept of the amyloidosis has emerged. It has been postulated that proteolytic cleavage of the precursor amyloidogenic protein leads to the formation of the peptides which assume the β-pleated conformation and the fibrillar structure characteristic of amyloid. According to this hypothesis the actual deposition of the amyloid fibers results from an imbalance between the production of the precursor protein and the ability to degrade it completely. This imbalance could be a result of a gene-dosage effect, as in Down's syndrome, or of overproduction of the amyloidogenic proteins resulting from antigenic stimulation (for example in experimental casein-induced or endotoxin-induced amyloidosis, or during chronic infections). It could also be due to gene mutation, as in some cases of familial amyloid polyneuropathy, or to alternative splicing of the mRNA. Another possibility is that as a result of age-associated changes or gene mutation the cells which process the amyloid precursor protein lose their ability to correctly degrade the amyloidogenic proteins.

We have identified some of the cells (the amyloidogenic protein processor cells) which are associated with the formation of the amyloid fibers in SDAT (Wisniewski et al. 1982; Merz et al. 1987). These cells appear to be pericytes, microglia, and as yet poorly defined cells in the walls of the large and medium-sized vessels. Irrespective of whether the brain reticuloendothelial cells (pericytes, microglia) are both producer and processor cells or only processor cells, the pathogenic events in plaque and vascular amyloid formation in AD/SDAT and unconventional virus infections appear to be similar to those observed in systemic amyloidosis. As indicated above, the intimate structural relationship between the amyloid fibers and the microglia-like cells suggests that these cells produce the amyloid fibers.

The data presented above suggest that amyloidosis of thh brain is the cause of cognitive pathology in AD. The differences between normal aged individuals and those affected by AD/SDAT appear to be quantitative and topographic (increase in density and extent of distribution; Kemper 1984; Ball et al. 1985; Hyman et al. 1986). Acceptance of the concept that AD/SDAT is a form of brain amyloidosis has both practical and theoretical consequences, i. e., if we want a laboratory diagnostic test we have to look for β-protein precursor proteins. The search for the amyloid-stimulating and -enhancing factors may lead us to the cause of AD. The treatment strategies must include a search for inhibition and/or activation of the AAAP-producing and/or -processing cells as well as methods which may help to remove the deposits of amyloid fibers.

Acknowledgments. The authors wish to thank Marjorie Agoglia for editorial and secretarial assistance.

---

*Supported in part by Grant No. AGO-4220 from the National Institute on Aging, NIH

References

Ball MJ, Hachinski V, Fox A, Kirshen AJ, Fisman M, Blume W, Kral VA, Fox H, Mersky H (1985) A new definition of Alzheimer's disease: a hippocampal dementia. Lancet 1: 14–16

Bobin SA, Styles J, Iqbal K, Miller DL, Wisniewski HM (1987) Alzheimer disease: structural homology between Alzheimer neuritic plaque core and cerebrovascular amyloid proteins. In preparation

Currie JR, Barcikowska M, Mehta P, Miller DL, Wisniewski HM (1987a) Immunocytochemical localization of the protein precursor of Alzheimer-related amyloid. In preparation

Currie JR, Chen MC, Bobin SA, Styles J, Miller DL, Kim KS, Wisniewski, HM (1987b) Immunochemical differences between cerebrovascular and neuritic plaque core amyloid proteins. In preparation

Divry, P (1934) De la nature de l'alteration fibrillaire d'Alzheimer. J Belge Neurol Psychiatr 34: 197–201

Glenner GG (1981) The bases of the staining of amyloid fibers: their physico-chemical nature and the mechanism of their dye-substrate interaction. Progr Histochem Cytochem 13: 1–37

Glenner GG, Wong CW (1984) Alzheimer's disease: initial report of the purification and characterization of a novel cerebrovascular amyloid protein. Biochem Biophys Res Commun 120: 885–890

Glenner GG, Wong CW (1986) The significance of cerebrovascular amyloid in Alzheimer's disease. International symposium on dementia and amyloid. Neuropathology (Suppl 3) 67–78

Goldgaber D, Lerman MI, McBride OW, Saffiotti U, Gajdusek DC (1987) Characterization and chromosomal localization of a cDNA encoding brain amyloid of Alzheimer's disease. Science, 235: 877–880

Grundke-Iqbal I, Iqbal K, Quinlan M, Wisniewski HM, Binder LI (1986a) Abnormal phosphorylation of the microtubule-associated protein (tau) in Alzheimer cytoskeletal pathology. Proc Natl Acad Sci USA 83: 4913–4917

Grundke-Iqbal I, Iqbal K, Quinlan M, Tung YC, Zaidi MS, Wisniewski HM (1986b) Microtubule-associated protein tau. J Biol Chem, 261: 6084–6089

Hyman BT, Van Hosen GW, Kromer LJ, Damasio AR (1986) Perforant pathway changes and the memory impairment of Alzheimer's disease. Ann Neurol, 20: 472–481

Iqbal K, Grundke-Iqbal I, Wisniewski HM (1987) Alzheimer's disease, microtubule and neurofilament proteins and axoplasmic flow. Lancet, 1: 102

Kang J, Lemaire HG, Unterbeck A, Salbaum JM, Masters CL, Grzeschik KH, Multhaup G, Beyreuther K, Muller-Hill B (1987) The precursor of Alzheimer's disease amyloid A4 protein resembles a cell-surface receptor. Nature 325: 733–736

Katzman R (1981) Early detection of senile dementia. Hosp Pract 16: 61–76

Kemper T (1984) Neuroanatomical and neuropathological changes in normal aging and in dementia. In Albert ML (ed) Clinical neurology of aging. Oxford University Press, New York, pp 9–52

Merz GS, Schwenk V, Schuller-Levis G, Gruca S, Wisniewski HM (1987) Isolation and characterization of macrophages from scrapie-infected mouse brain. Acta Neuropathol. (Berl), 72: 240–247

Mori H, Kondo J, Ihara Y (1987) Ubiquitin is a component of paired helical filaments in Alzheimer's disease. Science, 235: 1641–1644

Reisberg B, Ferris SH, DeLeon MJ (1985) Senile dementia of the Alzheimer type: diagnostic and differential diagnostic features with special reference to functional assessment staging. In: Traber J, Gispen WH (eds) Senile dementia of the Alzheimer type. Springer, Berlin Heidelberg New York, pp 18–37

Robakis NK, Ramakrishna N, Wolfe G, Wisniewski HM (1987a) Molecular cloning and characterization of a cDNA encoding the cerebrovascular and the neuritic plaque amyloid peptides. Proc Natl Acad Sci USA, 84: 4190–4194

Robakis NK, Wisniewski HM, Jenkins EC, Devine-Gage EA, Houck GE, Yao XL, Ramakrishna N, Wolfe G, Silverman WP, Brown WT (1987b) Chromosome 21q21 sublocalisation of gene encoding beta amyloid peptide in cerebral vessels and neuritic (senile) plaques of people with Alzheimer disease and Down syndrome. Lancet, 1: 384–385

Selkoe DJ, (1987) Deciphering Alzheimer's disease: the pace quickens. Trends Neurosci, 10: 181–184

Sternberger NH, Sternberger LA, Ulrich J (1985) Aberrant neurofilament phosphorylation in Alzheimer disease. Proc Natl Acad Sci USA, 82: 4274–4276

Terry RD, Hansen LA, DeTeresa R, Davies P, Tobias H, Katzman R (1987) Senile dementia of the Alzheimer type without neocortical neurofibillary tangles. J Neuropathol Exp Neurol, 46: 262–268

von Braunmuhl A (1957) Alterserkrankungen des Zentralnervensystems. Senile involution. Senile demenz. Alzheimerische Krankheit. In: Scholz W (ed) Nervensystem. Springer, Berlin Heidelberg New York, pp 22–539 (Handbuch der speziellen pathologischen Anatomie und Histologie, vol 13/1)

Wegelius O (1976) The place of amyloidosis in experimental and clinical medicine. In: Wegelius O, Pasternack A (eds) Amyloidosis. Academic, London, pp 1–13

Wisniewski H, Miller DL (1986) Morphology and biochemistry of abnormal fibrous proteins in Alzheimer's disease and senile dementia of the Alzheimer type (AD/SDAT). Neurobiol Aging 446–447

Wisniewski H, Soifer D (1979) Neurofibrillary pathology: current status and research perspectives. Mech Ageing Dev 9: 119–142

Wisniewski HM, Wrzolek M (1987) Pathogenesis of amyloid formation in Alzheimer disease, Down's syndrome and scrapie. Ciba Found Symp 135: in press

Wisniewski HM, Vorbrodt AW, Moretz RC, Lossinsky AS, Grundke-Iqbal I (1982) Pathogenesis of neuritic (senile) and amyloid plaque formation. In: Hoyer S (ed) The aging brain – physiological and pathophysiological aspects. Springer, Berlin Heidelberg New York, (Experimental brain research series, Suppl 5) World Health Organization (1986) Dementia in later life: research and action. WHO Report Series 730 pp 3–9

Wisniewski HM, Iqbal K, Grundke-Iqbal I, Rubenstein R, Wen GY, Merz PA, Kascsak R, Kristensson K (1986) Amyloid in Alzheimer's disease and unconventional viral infections. International symposium on dementia and amyloid. Neuropathology (Suppl 3) 87–94

Wisniewski HM, Rabe A, Wen GY, Wisniewski KE (1987a) Gene dose effect on early formation of neuritic plaques in Down syndrome (DS) (Abstract No 8). J Neurophathol Exp Neurol, 46: 334

Wisniewski HM, Rabe A, Wisniewski KE (1987b) Neuropathology and dementia in people with Down syndrome. In: Neurochemistry of aging, Banbury report. Cold Spring Harbor Laboratory (in press)

Wisniewski HM, Wen GY, Grundke-Iqbal I, Iqbal K, Mehta PD, Merz PA, Miller D, Currie J, Bobin SA, Robakis NK, Rabe A, Brown WT (1987c) Pathological, biochemical and genetic aspects of Alzheimer's disease in aged people and Down syndrome. In: Machleidt H (ed) Contributions of chemistry to health, Proceedings of the fifth CHEMRAWN conference, Heidelberg

World Health Organization (1986) Dementia in later life: research and action. WHO Report Series 730 pp 297–315

Immunological Markers and Neuropathological Lesions in Alzheimer's Disease

A. Pouplard-Barthelaix

Summary

Using direct immunofluorescence on 5-μm sections from frozen brain specimens obtained shortly after death, the different complement factors of the classical pathway (C1, C3, C4) were demonstrated in the brain amyloid lesions of four patients who had Alzheimer's disease.

Staining intensity appeared to depend on the kind of senile plaques. There was a predominance of C1q staining on plaques with a central amyloid core and on amyloid masses around the infiltrated vessels, and a predominance of C3 staining on neuritic plaques with no apparent central core. C1, C3, and C4 were constantly demonstrated in the infiltrated leptomeningeal and intracortical vessel walls. In addition, intensely stained round intraluminal cells were seen in one case and in another case, intense staining of some degenerating neurons; both were observed using anti-C3.

The few plaques of the brains of two senile patients without dementia used as controls also stained positively with anti-C1q and anti-C3, but no staining what so ever was detected in a case of Creutzfeldt-Jakob disease or in five other control caases. The three main classes of immunoglobulins (IgG, IgA, IgM) were found to coexist on the amyloid-infiltrated vessel walls.

From these findings, it could be postulated that immunological mechanisms are probably important in the appeerence of brain lesions in Alzheimer's disease and that the primary insult is located on the blood vessel walls.

Introduction

After the success of Glenner and Wong (1984a, b) in isolating the CVAP (cerebrovascular amyloid peptide), results from different teams working on the molecular biology of the β-amyloid protein (Wong CW et al., 1985), with the location of the gene of the precursor on chromosome 21 (Goldgaber et al., 1987; Kang et al., 1987) have shed light on the long-suspected relationship between Alzheimer's disease (AD) and Down's syndrome (DS). Nevertheless, much progress remains to be made to understand which environmental or pathogenic factors trigger the cellular and/or humoral mechanisms leading to the typical brain lesions of AD that exist by the 4th decade in virtually all DS cases.

DS patients have an immunodeficiency disorder and (Burgio et al., 1983; Smith and Warren, 1985) besides their high susceptibility to infection, autoimmune mechanisms, responsible for numerous pathological conditions, occur with increasing age. This, by analogy, has for a long time been the basis for the hypothesis of immunological mechanisms as a cause of Alzheimer's disease (Singh et al., 1987). The presence in AD sera of several kinds of circulating autoantibodies (Pouplard et al., 1983; Pouplard-Barthelaix et al., 1986; Singh and Fudenberg, 1986) lends further support to such a hypothesis, which would have to be verified by looking for immunological markers in the brain of patients with AD or senile dementia of the Alzheimer type (SDAT).

The use of frozen specimens obtained shortly after death, in addition to the classical neuropathological technique, has certainly allowed interesting observations in the field in the last few years. Results obtained in my studies strongly support the role of immunological mechanisms, whatever the initiating event, in the appearance of what is probably the most typical lesion of AD, amyloidosis.

Materials and Methods

The immunological study was conducted on post-mortem brain specimens obtained from 13 patients including four AD/SDAT patients, three patients with senile lesions (one with associated Hashimoto thyroiditis) but without apparent clinical dementia, one patient with Creutzfeldt-Jakob disease (CJD) and five controls who died from: a stroke, head injury, herpetic encephalitis, Parkinson's disease, and carcinomatous meningitis. In one case of AD with extensive amyloidosis, a brain biopsy obtained when the patient was alive was also examined.

All post-mortem tissues used (Ammon's horn, frontal and occipital cortex) were frozen in liquid nitrogen 2–6 h after death. After sampling the frozen specimens, brains were kept in 10% formaldehyde for the classical histopathological study. The immunohistochemical staining was realized on 5 μm frozen sections with antisera directed against several plasma proteins: albumin α-1-antitrypsine, C reactive Protein (CRP) P component, complement factors C1q, C3, C4, and heavy (γ, α, μ, δ) and light chains ($\varkappa$, λ) of human immunoglobulins. All of the different antisera except anti-P component were polyclonal, conjugated with fluorescein isothiocyanate (FITC), and so used in a direct immunofluorescent assay. The rabbit anti-P component was used in an indirect assay with FITC-conjugated goat anti-rabbit immunoglobulins. Monoclonal antisera directed against immunological cellular markers CD4, CD8, and Dr were used in the indirect assay with FITC-conjugated goat anti-mouse immunoglobulins.

To avoid non-specific reactions, only F (ab)'2 fragments of goat anti-human and anti-mouse immunoglobulins were used in this assay. Each antiserum was tested both on unfixed and fixed sections with three different 5-min fixations including 2% paraformaldehyde, acetone, and 20% (V/V) ice-cold methanol. One out of two sections from each specimen was kept for histological examination with Congo red staining. In addition, a double-labelling technique was performed on some sections: sections already stained with the fluorescent dye were counterstained with a 1% aqueous solution of Congo red.

Results

No staining was ever detected either on vessel walls or on senile plaques (SP) with several of the antisera: anti-CRP, anti-P component, anti α-1-antitrypsin and IgD. A faint and diffuse staining was often present around blood vessels on AD specimens as well as in control brains when stained with the anti-albumin antiserum, suggesting some post-mortem leakage of blood proteins.

Complement staining

With all antisera directed against the complement components C1q, C3 and C4, the amyloid deposits inside and around the vessel walls and in the SP were brightly stained. Differences in staining intensity were noticed among the four AD patients and these seemed to correlate with the severity of the lesions found through histopathological examination. They included intense C1q versus faint C3 staining on the amyloid core of SP and on the amyloid masses infiltrating the brain parenchyma around blood vessels (Fig. 1). In contrast, neuritic plaques without a central core were always brightly stained with anti-C3 (Fig. 2). In addition, in two cases, staining for C1q and C3 was detected on apparently extracellular tangles (Fig. 3).

Among the five control cases, a positive reaction for C3 and C4 was detected only in some leptomeningeal vessels in the carcinomatous meningitis case. This renders important the fact that all the occasional SP detected in the elderly control brain specimens were positive with both anti-C1q and/or anti-C3 antisera. We did not obtain any staining of the typical round plaques in the cerebellum of a case of CJD. However, a few typical neuritic plaques were detected in the hippocampus, providing results

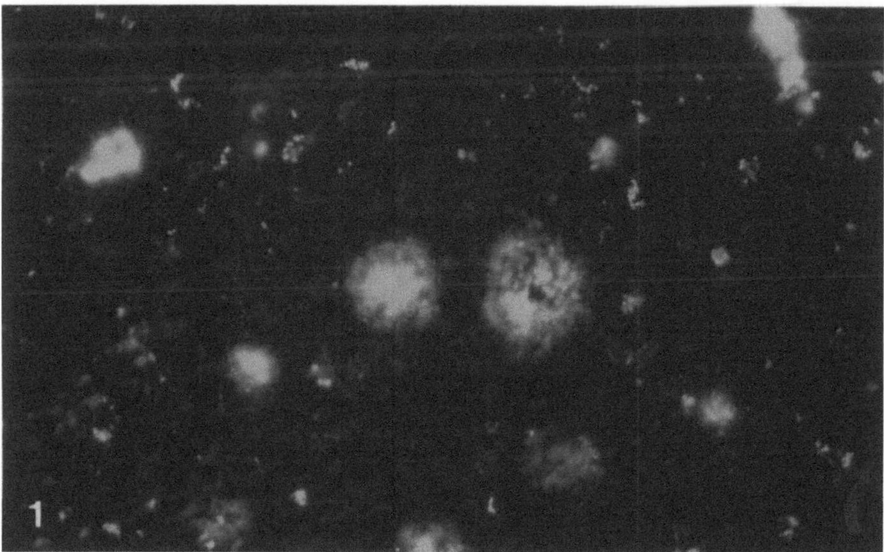

Fig 1. Direct IF: anti-C1q. SP with a central amyloid core and amyloid masses in the brain parenchyma are brightly stained (ATAB FITC goat anti-human C1q 1/50)

similar to those in the three other elderly patients. Fixation with acetone or methanol did not enhance the staining process and there was an important decrease under formadehyde fixation. This corresponds to the negative results reported using sections of classically fixed brain.

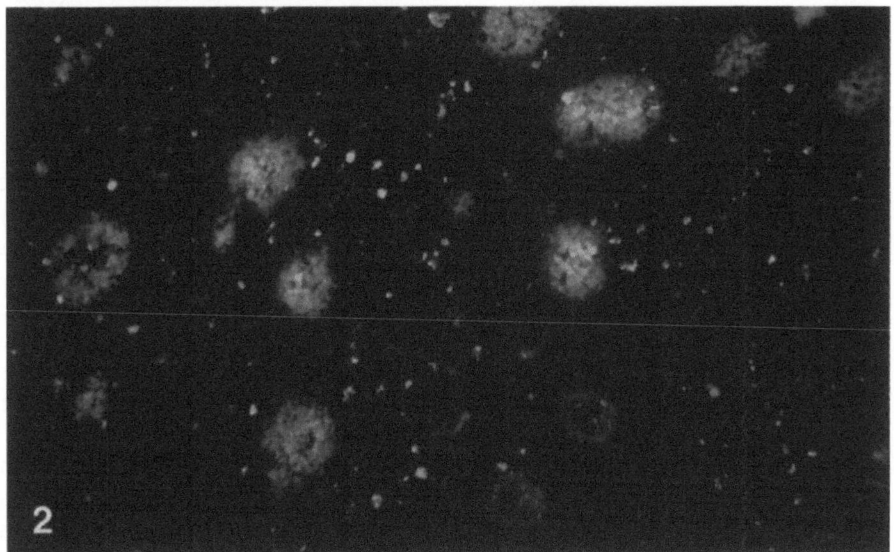

Fig. 2. Direct IF: anti-C3. Staining of neuritic SP without evident central amyloid core (ATAB FITC goat anti-human C3 1/50)

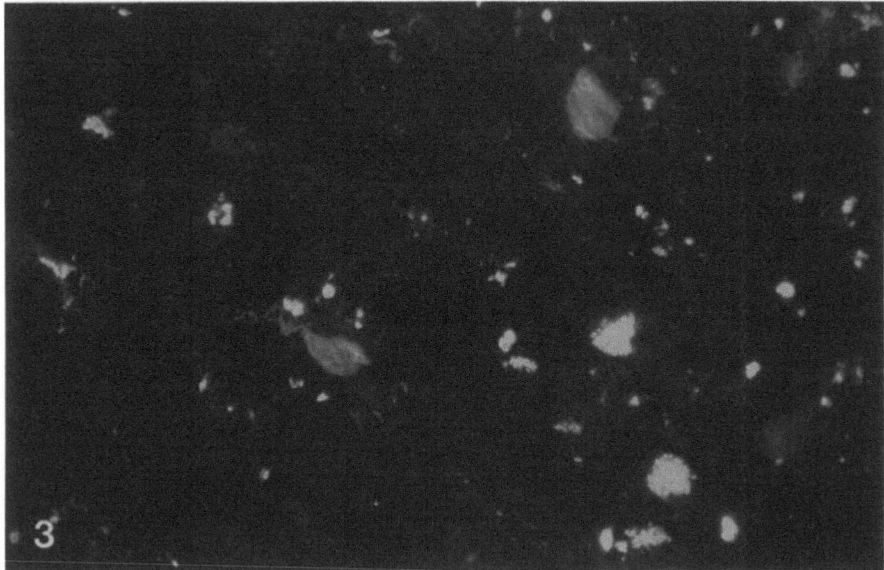

Fig. 3. Direct IF: anti-C3. Bright staining of apparently extracellular tangles

Immunoglobulins

The three main classes of human immunoglobulins – IgG, IgA and IgM – could be detected in the amyloid-infiltrated vessel wall (Fig. 4). In most vessels, positive results were obtained with at least two of the three antisera. IgG and IgM were more frequently detected than IgA. No brightness similar to that obtained with the anti-complement components was obtained either on amyloid masses around blood vessels or on the classical SP. The faint and diffuse staining obtained with the anti-IgG was not very different from that obtained with anti-albumin. In only one case, although faint, were SP clearly detected with the anti-IgA.

The amyloid plaques and vessels in the CJD brain did not show any staining, and neither did the five control brains. In contrast, in all three elderly patients without dementia, brightly stained small pericapillary deposits were demonstrated. They were predominantly of the IgA and IgM classes. In addition, small arteries were detected with walls heavily stained with one of the three antisera.

Cellular markers

With anti-CD4 and -CD8, occasional round positive cells, located either in the lumen or in the wall of some vessels, were seen; their presence did not seem to correlate with evident amyloid deposits. CD8-positive cells were more numerous in the case of associated Hashimoto thyroiditis. Obviously positive results were obtained with three different monoclonal anti-Dr antisera, and better results were seen on unfixed sections and sections fixed with ice-cold methanol.

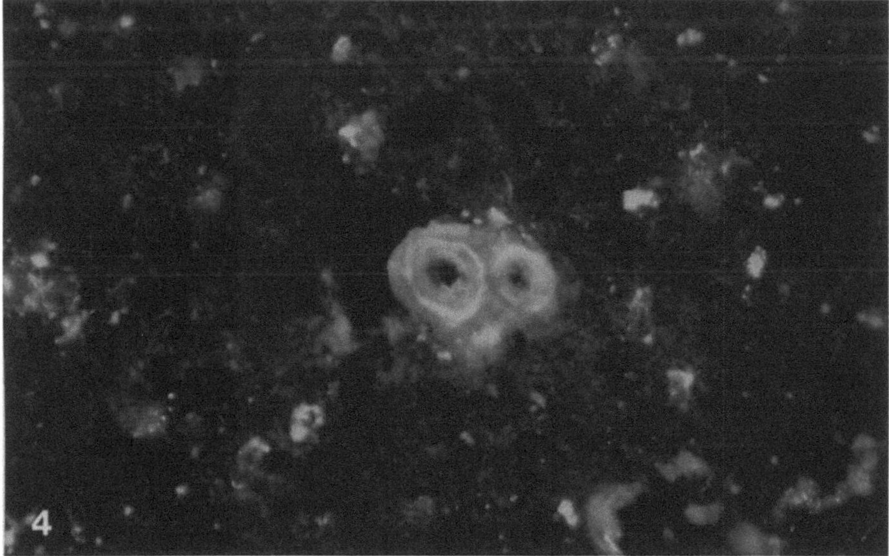

Fig. 4. Direct IF: anti-IgG. The walls of two infiltrated amyloid vessels are heavily stained (Biosys-F(ab)'2 anti-human γ 1/50)

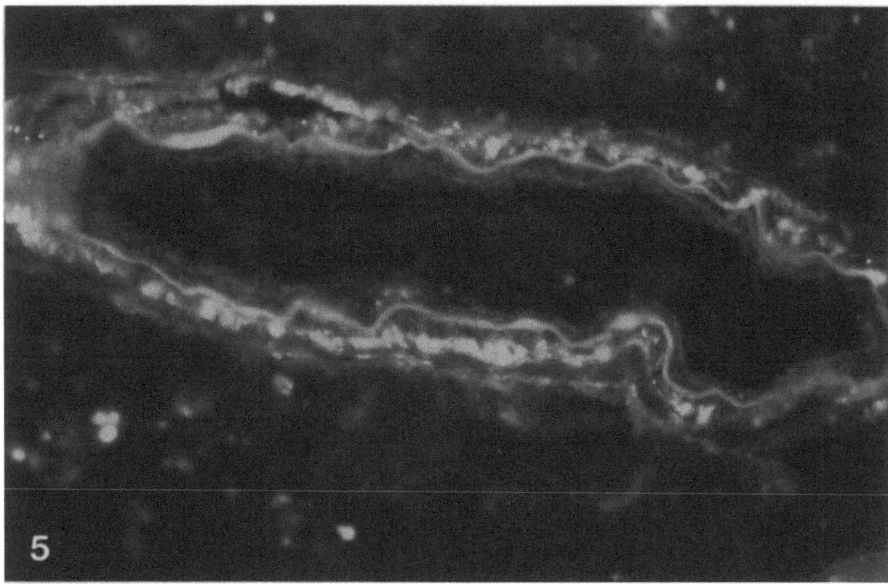

Fig. 5. Indirect IF staining with mouse monoclonal anti-Dr (Dakopatts) counterstain with FITC F(ab)'2 fragments of sheep anti-mouse immunoglobulins (silenus). The wall of a large vessel shows intense staining

Different patterns could be observed depending on brain specimens. For all four AD cases, positive staining, lying predominantly on some endothelial cells and on some cells lining the vessel wall that looked like pericytes, could be detected on large and medium size vessels (Fig. 5). The most intense staining was found in the biopsy obtained from the case of AD with extensive amyloidosis. A light but clear staining was often present on SP, more evidently on neuritic SP with occasional small positive rings corresponding to infiltrating "microglial" cells. In addition, similar sparse cells were seen close to some degenerating neurons, as demonstrated in double-stained sections. In three cases, including the elderly patient with Hashimoto thyroiditis, positive cells could be detected in the lumen of small vessels (Fig. 6) with some of the cells streaming out inside the brain parenchyma. In all four cases of AD/SDAT and in the three elderly patients, the lumen of numerous microcapillaries was brightly lined.

Discussion

Since the first report by Ishii et al. (1975), the presence of immunoglobulins in the amyloid deposits of brains of patients with AD has been documented, but with some controversial results (Ishii and Haga, 1976; Powers et al., 1981). Under the conventional light microscope we found the presence of immunoglobulins inside the SP difficult to ascertain in contrast to their obvious presence inside the amyloid deposits of the vessel wall.

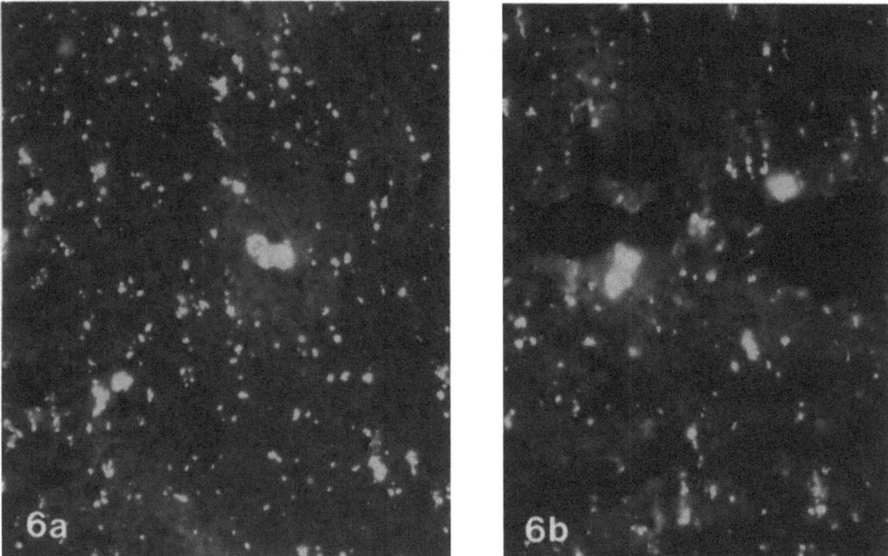

Fig. 6. Indirect IF staining with mouse monoclonal anti-Dr. Positive cells in the lumen of a vessel (a) looking as if they are streaming out in brain parenchyma (b)

Concerning the complement components, similar results have been reported by different authors with evidence of the first components of the classical pathway – C1q, C4, C3 – both in the cerebrovascular and SP deposits, (Eikelenboom and Stam, 1982; Ishii and Haga, 1983, 1984). Their presence on the amyloid fibrils was confirmed by Ishii at the electron microscopic level. Evidence indicates that the presence of complement components is not due to a simple adsorption which is secondary to change in the blood-brain barrier or to post-mortem extravasation. In fact the best results in our study were obtained on a brain biopsy which was frozen immediately after death in the surgical room. Moreover, results obtained with different specimens frozen at various intervals after death tend to show that post-mortem autolysis would end up with barely significant results.

Activation of the complement pathway can be triggered by many substances (Linder et al., 1979; Pouplard-Barthelaix et al., 1986). The presence of complement components together with immunoglobulins, at least on the vascular deposits, may indicate antigen antibody complexes; if this is the case we will have to explain the lack of reactivity obtained by others with antisera against the last components of the pathway C5/C9 and the poor detection of immunoglobulins inside the SP. Active phagocytosis of such immune complexes could be one explanation.

The presence of C1q suggests an activation of the classical pathway, but the predominant C3 staining obtained in one case with numerous neuritic plaques, together with some IgA staining of the same plaques, could suggest that at least in some cases the activation can occur through the alternate pathway. Comparison of the staining obtained for C1q and C3 with Congo red, either on adjacent sections or in double-staining experiments, tends to show that whatever the physiological significance, the use of anti-C1q and anti-C3 could allow a rapid and sensitive detection of amyloid deposits in post-mortem brain and biopsy specimens.

In addition to the complement factors, detection of increased expression of Dr antigen favours a role for active immunological mechanisms in AD. HLA Dr or class II cell surface antigens of the major histocompatibility complex (MHC) must be present on the surface of the target cell together with the antigen to allow the recognition of the antigen by the T cell. The normal brain is considered an immunologically privileged site. Dr antigens have been detected only in 1%–2% of cells (De Tribolet et al., 1984). However, an increase in their expression could be demonstrated under treatment with some lymphokines such as interferon gamma (IFNγ) (Wong GH et al., 1985). In recent years it has been suggested that an increased expression of Dr on the target cell might be associated with some autoimmune conditions (Hashimoto and type I diabetes mellitus), and that the recognition of the autoantigen together with the Dr epitope by the T cells may lead to cellular death. Taking this hypothesis, the finding of an abnormal expression of Dr in the AD-affected brain would favour a role for autoimmune mechanisms and our results have recently been confirmed (McGeer et al. 1987). Moreover, the detection of these mechanisms on the surface of the vessel would suggest that, whatever the antigen, modified brain antigen or external antigen, the primary event of AD and/or of the genesis of SP takes place in brain capillaries. Such a localisation of an immunological attack fits Miyakawa's assumption, based on extensive electron microscopic studies, that in most AD patients, each SP contains at least one microvessel (Miyakawa et al., 1982; Miyakawa et al., 1986), with an altered blood-brain barrier (Alafuzoff et al., 1987; Pouplard-Barthelaix et al., 1986; Wisniewski and Koslowski, 1982) and that circulating antibodies against brain microvessels are detected. The expression of a foreign or modified self antigen on the brain vessel would not be surprising because in a "privileged" tissue devoid of classical lymphatic drainage, blood certainly represents the normal way for antigens to reach the immunological system.

Predominant humoral immunological mechanisms acting at the microvessel level also fit with Glenner's vascular hypothesis of AD based on molecular results for the β-amyloid protein and its circulating precursor (Glenner et al., 1986).

The presence of complement components inside the amyloid deposits raises the question of their role in the local processing of the cerebral amyloid precursor, since these components could be considered amongst the most potent serine proteases and since proteolysis has been demonstrated to be one of the major mechanisms in amyloid fibril formation (Glenner 1980); therefore, it will be interesting to look for β-amyloid or its precursor as a potentially modified self antigen.

An autoimmune reaction constituting the basis of brain lesions in DS would not be surprising: DS patients are known to develop a variety of autoimmune disorders with autoantibodies, thyroid autoimmunity being the predominant feature. DS patients' progressive immune deficiency is certainly complex and is not yet elucidated. These patients have an increased sensitivity to interferon, not only to the antiviral effect, and this has been explained with the location of the receptor gene on the long arm of chromosome 21. An increase in Dr expression secondary to a hypersensitivity to IFN-γ could be an important factor that renders DS patients susceptible to the development of autoimmune pathology. Premature ageing is considered one of the most characteristic features of DS. A deterioration of cellular immunity with an increase of circulating autoantibodies is known to occur during ageing (Vissin and Dirven, 1987), and an increased sensitivity to interferon has been described in AD patients (Weinreb and Burskirk, 1987).

In spite of the recent location on chromosome 21 both of the β-amyloid precursor gene (Robakis et al., 1987) and of the gene of the autosomal dominant form of the disease (familial Alzheimer's disease, FAD) (Van Broeckhoven et al., 1987), none of the genetic evidence clearly identifies the possible cause of AD at the moment. Complex interactions between several gene products of chromosome 21 or of other chromosomes could be taken into consideration as could immunological mechanisms, which may interfere as primary or secondary events. An immunological hypothesis is not exclusive and it may be that numerous factors, including pathogens, contribute to the generation of autoantibodies in susceptible individuals.

References

Alafuzoff I, Adolfsson R, Grundke-Iqbal I, Windblad B (1987) Blood brain barrier in Azheimer's dementia and in non demented elderly. Acta Neuropathol. (Berlin) 73: 160–166

Burgio GR, Ugazio A, Nespoli L, Maccario R (1983) Down's syndrome: a model of immunodeficiency. Birth Defects 19: 325–327

De Tribolet N, Hamou MF, Mach JP, Carrel S, Schreyer M (1984) Demonstration of HLA-Dr antigens in normal human brain. J Neurol Neurosurg Psychiatr 47: 417–418

Eikelenboom P, Stam FC (1982) Immunoglobulins and complement factors in senile plaques. Acta Neuropathol (Berlin) 57: 239–242

Glenner GG (1980) Amyloid deposits and amyloidosis: the β fibrilloses. New Engl J Med 302: 1283–1292, 1333–1343

Glenner GG, Wong W (1984a) Alzheimer's disease: initial report of the purification and characterization of novel cerebrovascular amyloid protein. Biochem Biophys Res Commun 120: 885–890

Glenner GG, Wong W (1984b) Alzheimer's disease and Down's syndrome: sharing of a unique cerebrovascular amyloid fibril protein. Biochem Biophys Res Commun 122: 1131–1135

Glenner GG, Wong CW, Quaranta V, Eanes ED (1986) The amyloid deposits in Alzheimer's disease: their nature and pathogenesis. Appl Pathol 83: 7908–7912

Goldgaber D, Lerman MI, McBride OW, Saffiotti U, Gadjdusek DC (1987) Characterization of a c DNA encoding brain amyloid of Alzheimer's disease. Science 235: 877–880

Ihara Y, Kurizaki H, Nukina N, Sugita H, Toyokura Y, Ebara C (1981) Presence of immunoglobulin light chain in the core of senile plaques – an unlabelled antibody peroxidase-antiperoxydase study. Neurological Medicine (Japan) 15: 292–295

Ishii T, Haga S, Shimizu F (1975) Identification of components of immunoglobulins in senile plaques by means of fluorescent antibody technique. Acta Neuropathol (Berlin) 32: 157–162

Ishii T, Haga S (1976) Immunoelectro microscopic localization of immunoglobulins in amyloid fibrils of senile plaques. Acta Neuropathol (Berlin) 36: 243–249

Ishii T, Haga S (1983) The presence of immunoglobulins and complements in senile plaques: an immunofluorescent study. Neuropathology (Japan) 4: 31–36

Ishii T, Haga S (1984) Immunoelectro microscopic localization of complements in amyloid fibrils of senile plaques. Acta Neuropathol (Berlin) 63: 296–300

Kang J, Lemaire HG, Unter-Beck A, Salbaum JM, Masters CI, Grzeschik KH, Multhaup G, Beyreuther K, Muller Hill B (1987) The precursor of Alzheimer's disease – amyloid A4 protein resembles a cell surface receptor. Nature 325: 733–736

Linder E, Lehto VP, Stenman S (1979) Activation of complement by cytoskeletal intermediate filaments. Nature 278: 176–178

McGeer PL, Itagaki S, Tago H, McGeer EG (1987) Reactive microglia in patients with senile dementia of the Alzheimer type are positive for the histocompatibility glycoprotein HLA- Dr. Neuroscience Letters 79: 195–200

Miyakawa T, Shimoji A, Kuramoto R, Higuchi Y (1982) The relationship between senile plaques and cerebral blood vessels in Alzheimer's disease and senile dementia – morphological mechanism of senile plaque production. Virchows Arch (Cell Pathol) 40: 121–129

Miyakawa T, Katsuragi S, Watanabe K, Shimoji A, Ikeuchi Y (1986) Ultrastructural studies of amyloid fibrils and senile plaques in human brain. Acta Neuropathol 70: 202–208

Pouplard A, Emile J, Vincent-Pineau F (1983) Autoanticorps circulants anti-cellules à Prolactine de l'hypophyse humaine et maladie d'Alzheimer. Rev Neurol 139: 187–191

Pouplard-Barthelaix A, Dubas F, Jabbour W, Maher I, Emile J (1986) An immunological view on the etiology and pathogenesis of Alzheimer's disease. In: A Bes, (Ed). Senile dementia early detection. John Libbey Eurotext, Paris, pp 216–222

Pouplard-Barthelaix A, Jabbour W, Berger F, Delamarche C, Gallard L, Emile J: Altered blood brain barrier functions in Alzheimer's disease: an immunological study (submitted)

Powers JM, Schlaepfer WW, Willingham ML, Hall BJ (1981) An immunoperoxidase study of senile cerebral amyloidosis with pathogenetic considerations. J Neuropathol Exp Neurol 40: 592–612

Robakis NK, Wisniewski HM, Jewkins EC, Devine-Gage EA, Houck GE, Yao XL, Ramakrishna N, Wolfe G, Silverman WP, Brown WT (1987) Chromosome 21q21 sublocalisation of gene encoding β amyloid peptide in cerebral vessels and neuritic (senile) plaques of people with Alzheimer's disease and Down's syndrome. Lancet, 385

Singh VK, Fudenberg HH (1986) Detection of brain autoantibodies in the serum of patients with Alzheimer's disease but no Down's syndrome. Immunol Lett 12: 277–280

Singh VK, Fudenberg HH, Brown FR (1987) Immunologic dysfunction: simultaneous study of Alzheimer's and older Down's patients. Mech Ageing Develop 37: 257–264

Smith GF, Warren ST (1985) The biology of Down's syndrome. Ann NY Acad Sci 450: 19

Van Broeckhoven C, Genthe AM, Vandenberghe A, Horsthemke B, Backhovens H, Raeymaekers P, Van Hul W, Wehnert A, Gheuens J, Cras P, Bruyland M, Martin JJ, Salbaum M, Multhaup G, Masters CL, Beyreuther K, Gurling HMD, Mullan MJ, Holland A, Barton A, Irving N, Williamson R, Richards SJ, Hardy JA (1987) Failure of familial Alzheimer's disease to segregate with the A4-amyloid gene in several European families. Nature 329: 153–155

Vissin GA, Dirven CI (1987) Deterioration of cellular immunity during aging. Cell Immunol 108: 323–324

Weinreb HJ, Burskirk DR (1987) Enhanced lymphocyte interferon sensitivity in Alzheimer's disease. J Am Geriatr Soc 35: 1–85

Wisniewski HM, Koslowski P (1982) Evidence for blood brain barrier changes in senile dementia of the Alzheimer type (SDAT). Ann NY Acad Sci 396: 119–129

Wong GH, Bartlett PF, Clark Lewis I, McKimm-Breschkin JL, Schrader JW (1985) Interferon alpha induces expression of H2 and Ia antigen on brain cells. J Neuroimmunol 7: 255–278

Wong CW, Quaranta WV, Glenner GR (1985) Neuritic plaques and cerebrovascular amyloid in Alzheimer's disease are antigenically related. Proc Natl Acad Sci USA 82: 8729–8732

Presence of Immunoglobulins and Complements in the Amyloid Plaques in the Brain of Patients with Alzheimer's Disease

T. Ishii, S. Haga, and *F. Kametani*

Summary

The presence of immunoglobulins and complement factors in the amyloid in senile plaques in the brain of six patients with Alzheimer's disease has been demonstrated by means of immunofluorescence, immunoperoxidase, or the avitin-biotin complex immunoperoxidase (ABC) method.

A positive immunohistochemical reaction of senile plaques was noted with anti-IgG antibody. Not all the senile plaques showed the positive reaction to anti-IgG antibody. The reason for the negative reactions is not known, but antigenic sites of immunoglobulins were probably partially masked by the subsequent activation of complement cascades. Immunohistochemistry revealed that the complements C1q, C4, and C3 were on the amyloid fibrils of senile plaques, but results for complements C5–C9 were consistently negative. Other serum components such as albumin, prealbumin, IgA, IgM, CRP (C-reactive protein), and β_2-microglobulin were not found in the amyloid of senile plaques, nor were other factors related to the immunological response of the central nervous system such as HLA, B cells, OKB2, granulocytes, leukocytes, or fibronectin.

If the presence of C1q and C3 in the amyloid of senile plaques is an immune reaction triggered by an immune complex, this might explain the tissue damage surrounding the amyloid fibrils, i.e., the senile plaque formation.

Introduction

The deposition of amyloid plaques is considered one of the most characteristic chemical and pathological hallmarks in the brain of patients with Alzheimer's disease (Alzheimer 1907) and the number of these amyloid plaques seems to correlate with the degree of dementia (Blessed et al. 1968). Chemical analysis of the amyloid in the senile plaques in the brains both of patients with Alzheimer's disease and of those with Down's syndrome disclosed a unique polypeptide, the amino acid sequence of which has no homology with the known polypeptides (Glenner and Wong 1984; Masters et al. 1985). Thee gene encoding the protein is localized on chromosome 21 (Goldgaber et al. 1987; Kang et al. 1987; Robakis et al. 1987; St George-Hyslop et al. 1987; Tanzi et al. 1987).

Another aspect of these amyloid deposits in the brain of patients with Alzheimer's disease is the presence of immunoglobulins and complements. Since our first reports

18   T. Ishii et al.

(Ishii et al. 1975; Ishii and Haga 1976a), the presence of immunoglobulins in the amyloid in senile plaques has been confirmed immunohistochemically by Ihara et al. (1981), Powers et al. (1981), and Eikelenboom and Stam (1982).

Immunoperoxidase histochemistry has disclosed the presence of the complements C1q, C3, and C4 in senile plaques (Eikelenboom and Stam 1982; Ishii and Haga 1983b). An immunoelectron microscopic study has also confirmed that these complements are localized on the amyloid fibrils and that no other tissue elements were stained (Ishii and Haga 1984a). These findings suggest the operation of immunological mechanisms in the pathogenesis of the amyloid plaques in the brain of patients with Alzheimer's disease. Immunoblot analysis of emulsions of such brains has also disclosed the presence of complements (see below). A monoclonal antibody against microglia, which has been raised recently in our institute, stains macrophages and is seemingly active in the production, or phagocytosis, of amyloid in the Alzheimer-affected brain (Haga et al. 1986).

However, there are reports that have shown the presence of other serum components such as albumin or prealbumin, together with immunoglobulins and complements, in brain tissue from patients with Alzheimer's disease and that have interpreted the presence of immunoglobulins and complements in the amyloid in senile plaques as being merely a reflection of the diffusion of the serum proteins from the blood.

To explore the possibility of a fortuitous adsorption of these immunoglobulins and complements by the amyloid in senile plaques, we have examined the tissue of the brain immunohistochemically with a wide variety of antibodies against serum components and related proteins. Our results have confirmed that only immunoglobulins and the complements C1q, C4, and C3 are present in the amyloid in senile plaques, though serum proteins such as albumin, IgM, and IgA are found distributed perivascularly in some patients with Alzheimer's disease as well as in the brains of nondemented age-matched controls.

Materials and Methods

The brains of six patients with histologically and clinically verified Alzheimer's disease were used. Five control brains were also examined. These cases, with some clinicopathologic details, are presented in Table 1.

Table 1. Clinico-pathological findings in six patients with Alzheimer's disease

Case	Clinico-pathological diagnosis	Age/Sex	Brain weight (g)	Neuropathology
K.T.	AD	63 F	1150	SP, ANT, AA
K.T.	AD	61 F	755	SP, ANT, AA
K.I.	SDAT	88 M	1170	SP, ANT, AA
E.T.	SDAT	86 F	1110	SP, ANT, AA
H.K.	SDAT	74 F	1115	SP, ANT
I.F.	SDAT	89 F	1055	SP, ANT

AD, Alzheimer's disease; SDAT, senile dementia of the Alzheimer type; SP, senile plaque; ANT, Alzheimer's neurofibrillary tangle; AA, amyloid angiopathy

Histochemistry

Cryostat sections from the frontal cortex and the hippocampus were stained using the indirect immunofluorescence, immunoperoxidase, and avitin-biotin complex immunoperoxidase (ABC) techniques, as have been described elsewhere (Ishii et al. 1975; Ishii and Haga 1984a). Antibody binding was observed under a fluorescent microscope or visualized in a diaminobenzidine (DAB) solution (0.05 M Tris/0.05% DAB/0.01% H_2O_2, pH 7.6). For light microscopic observations, the sections were counterstained with dilute hematoxylin. For electron microscopy the sections on slides were fixed with 2% glutaraldehyde after the DAB reaction, postfixed with 1% OsO_4, dehydrated, and embedded in epon. After hardening of the resin, the slides were removed and the tissue on the surface of the resin was cut. The ultrathin sections, stained or unstained, were observed under a JEM 200CX electron microscope at 80 kV. Control sections, for the first step, were treated with nonimmunized mouse serum (1:20) and mouse immunoglobulins (1:20). Some brain tissue slices were digested with 0.1% trypsin at 37°C for 5 min before incubation with primary antisera.

Electrophoresis and Western Blotting

The tissue was homogenized in 5 volumes of 62.5 mM Tris-HCl, pH 6.8, containing 2.3% sodium dodecyl sulfate (SDS) and 5% 2-mercaptoethanol. The homogenate was then centrifuged at 18000 × g for 35 min and the resultant supernatant was used for electrophoresis. The SDS-polyacrylamide gel electrophoresis was run in a 4%–17% linear-gradient gel slab (Laemmli 1970). After electrophoresis, the proteins were transferred from the gel to a nitrocellulose sheet by electrophoresis as described by Towbin et al. (1979). The nitrocellulose sheet was incubated with the monoclonal antibody (1:100 dilution) at 4°C for 16 h and the protein spot was visualized by means of the ABC technique.

Results

Immunohistochemical reactions of the amyloid in senile plaques toward the antibodies against serum proteins are summarized in Table 2, and toward the antibodies against some other proteins related to the immunological response of the CNS in Table 3.

Positive immunohistochemical reaction of the amyloid in senile plaques was noted with anti-IgG (Fig. 1). Not all the senile plaques showed the positive reaction to anti-IgG antibody. Amyloid deposits in the walls of small blood vessels (amyloid angiopathy) and those in the meninges were beautifully stained. Further, all these amyloid deposits were stained with the anticomplements C1q, C3, and C4, with the immunoperoxidase, and with the ABC method (Fig. 2). However, anti-C5 through C9 antibodies never showed a positive reaction with the amyloid in senile plaques. Other serum components such as albumin, prealbumin, IgA, IgM, C-reactive protein, and β_2-microglobulin (Table 2) were not found in the amyloid of senile plaques, and neither were other proteins related to the immunological response of the CNS such as human leukocyte antigen (HLA), B cells, OKB2, granulocytes, leukocytes, or fibronectin (Table 3). Occasionally, albumin, IgM, and IgA were found around the small blood vessels, but not on the amyloid fibrils of senile plaques (Fig. 3).

Immunoelectron microscopy demonstrated that only the amyloid fibrils among tissue elements became electron dense and thick with the DAB reaction product of the HRP anticomplement C1q antibody complex (Fig. 4). Neurofilaments in the axons and Alzheimer's neurofibrillary tangles in the nerve cells and in the axons did not become electron dense. Glial filaments and degenerated neuronal processes also showed no reaction products. At times we observed macrophages and the walls of

Table 2. Immunohistochemical reactions of the amyloid in senile plaques toward the antibodies against serum proteins

Primary antisera	Company	Method	Senile plaques	Perivascular space
Antihuman C1q (goat)	Cappel	IP, IF	++	−
Antihuman C4 (goat)	Miles	IP, IF	++	−
Antihuman C3 (goat)	Miles	IP, IF	+	−
Antihuman C5 (goat)	Miles	IP, IF	−	−
Antihuman C6 (goat)	Miles	IP	−	−
Antihuman C7 (goat)	Miles	IP	−	−
Antihuman C8 (goat)	Miles	IP	−	−
Antihuman C9 (goat)	Cappel	IP	−	−
Antihuman properdin (goat)	Miles	IP	−	−
Antihuman albumin (rabbit)	Cappel	IP, IF	−	+
Antihuman IgA (M)	BRL	IF	−	+
Antihuman IgD (M)	BRL	IF	−	±
Antihuman IgE (M)	BRL	IF	−	± ∼ +
Antihuman IgG (rabbit)	Cappel	IP, IF	+, −	+
Antihuman IgM (rabbit)	Cappel	IP, IF	−	+
Antihuman prealbumin (rabbit)	DAKO	IF	−	−
Antihuman CRP (goat)	Miles	IP	−	−
Antihuman P component (rabbit)	DAKO	IP	+	−
Antihuman β_2-microglobulin (M)	Sera lab	IF	−	−
Antihuman fibrinogen (goat)	E.Y.	IP	−	++

M, monoclonal antibody; CRP, C-reactive protein; IP, immunoperoxidase method; IF, immunofluorescent method

Table 3. Immunohistochemical reactions of the amyloid in senile plaques toward some proteins related to the immunological response of the CNS

Primary antisera	Company	Method	Senile plaques
Antihuman lysozyme (rabbit)	DAKO	IF	−
Antihuman HLA (M)	BRL	IF	−
Antihuman B cell (M)	Sera lab	IF	−
Antihuman OKB2 (M)	Ortho-mune	IP	−
Antihuman granulocyte (M)	Sera lab	IF	−
Antihuman leukocyte (M)	BRL	IF	−
Antihuman neuron (M)	Sera lab	IF	−
Antihuman fibronectin (M)	Sera lab	IF	−

IF, immunofluorescent method; IP, immunoperoxidase method

small blood vessels near the amyloid in senile plaques. The immunostaining of macrophages with a monoclonal antimacrophage antibody raised recently in our laboratory disclosed that many macrophages with long processes were located near the senile plaques or were even in close contact with the amyloid (Fig. 5).

Figure 6 illustrates the production or phagocytosis of amyloid fibrils near the cytoplasmic membrane of macrophages.

Immunoblot analysis of the brain emulsion showed the presence of a positive spot against the anticomplement C1q antibody (Fig. 7).

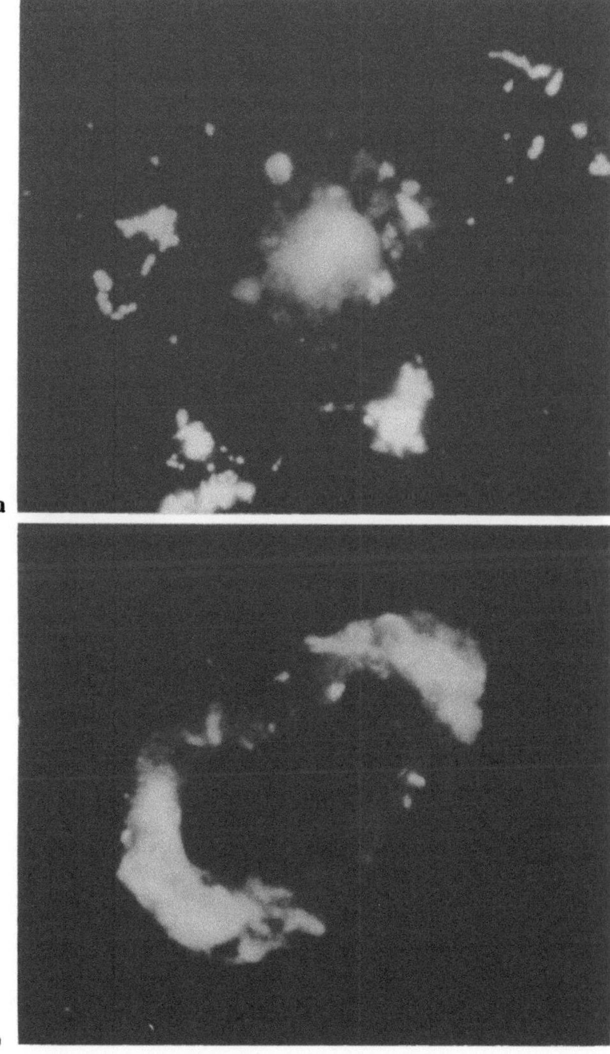

Fig. 1a, b. a Positive immunofluorescence of a senile plaque core, and **b** of an amyloid angiopathy, with an anti-IgG antibody

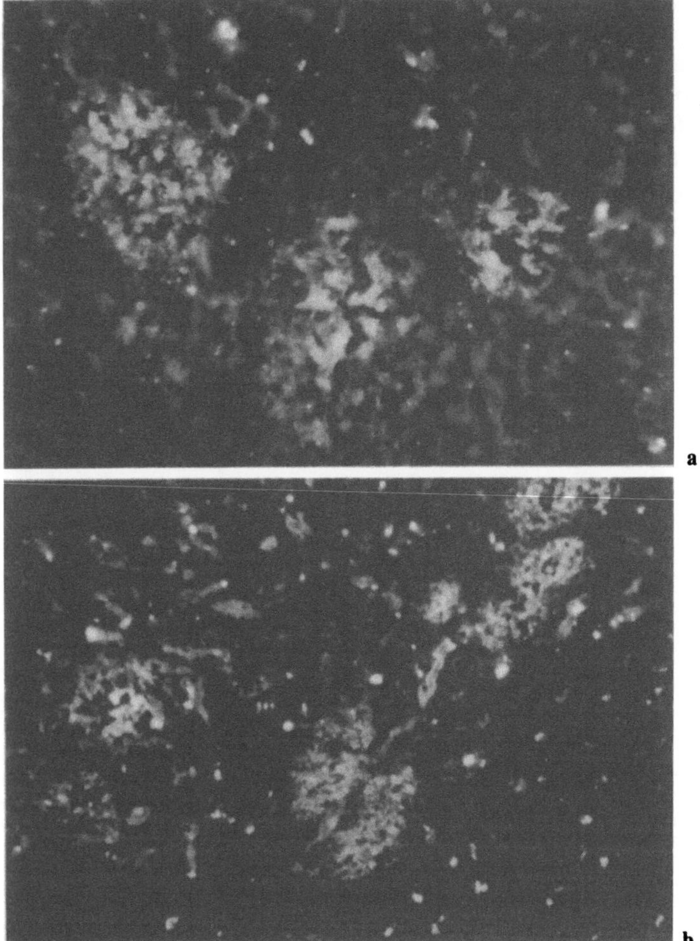

Fig. 2a, b. **a** Positive immunofluorescence of senile plaques with an anti-C1q, and **b** with an anti-C4 antibody

Discussion

There are two possible explainations for the presence of IgG and complements in the amyloid plaques of the brain in patients with Alzheimer's disease, i.e., a physical adsorption of complements to amyloid or an immunological binding. There is considerable circumstantial evidence that the presence of the complements proved here is due to a biological binding. The change in the permeability of the blood-brain barrier (Wisniewski and Kozlowski 1982; Alafuzoff et al. 1987), which implements the complements into the CNS may be an indication of the immune response in the CNS. Many serum components other than the complements, such as albumin or a large molecule like IgM, proved negative in amyloid plaques, though they were found

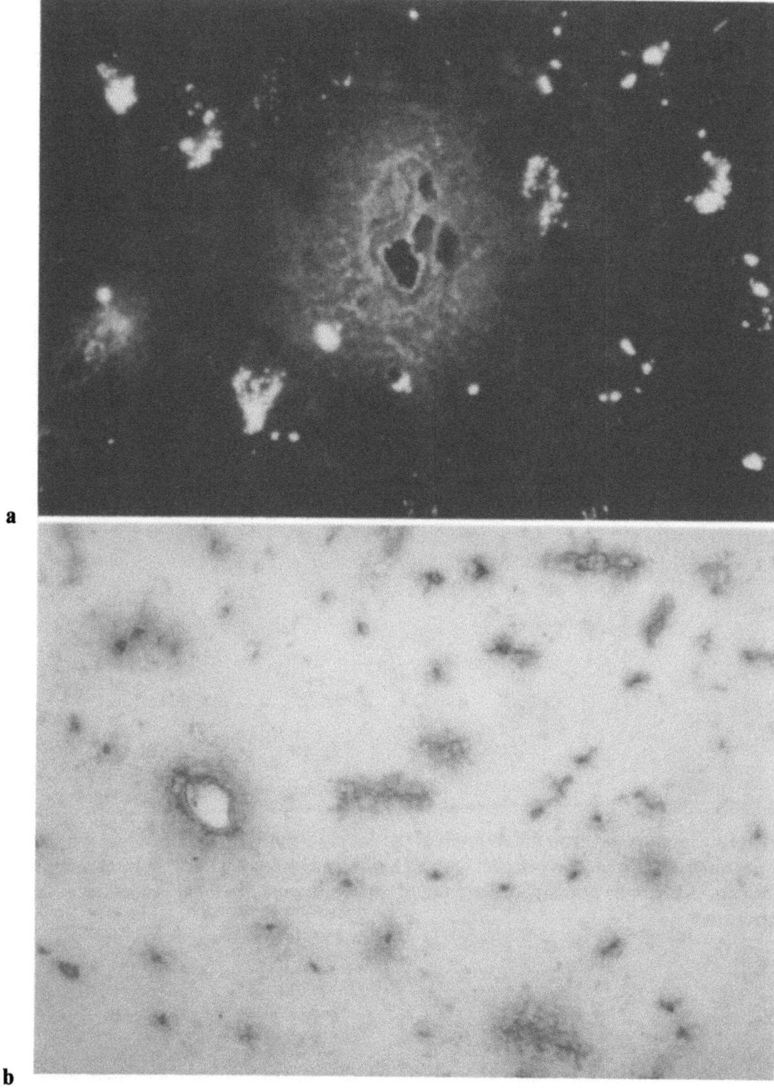

Fig. 3a, b. a Positive immunofluorescence and immunoperoxidase reaction with an anti-IgA antibody, and **b** with an antifibrinogen antibody, around a small blood vessel

perivascularly in the Alzheimer-affected brain as well as in those of age-matched controls. Furthermore, there is a definite pattern in the reactions with anticomplement antisera in our study, i. e., a very strong reaction with anti-C1q and C4, a weaker one with C3, and a consistently negative one with C5 through C9. Electron microscopy of amyloid stained with anticomplement C1q disclosed thickened fibrils but no trace of a reaction product between the fibrils, nor any on the other tissue elements

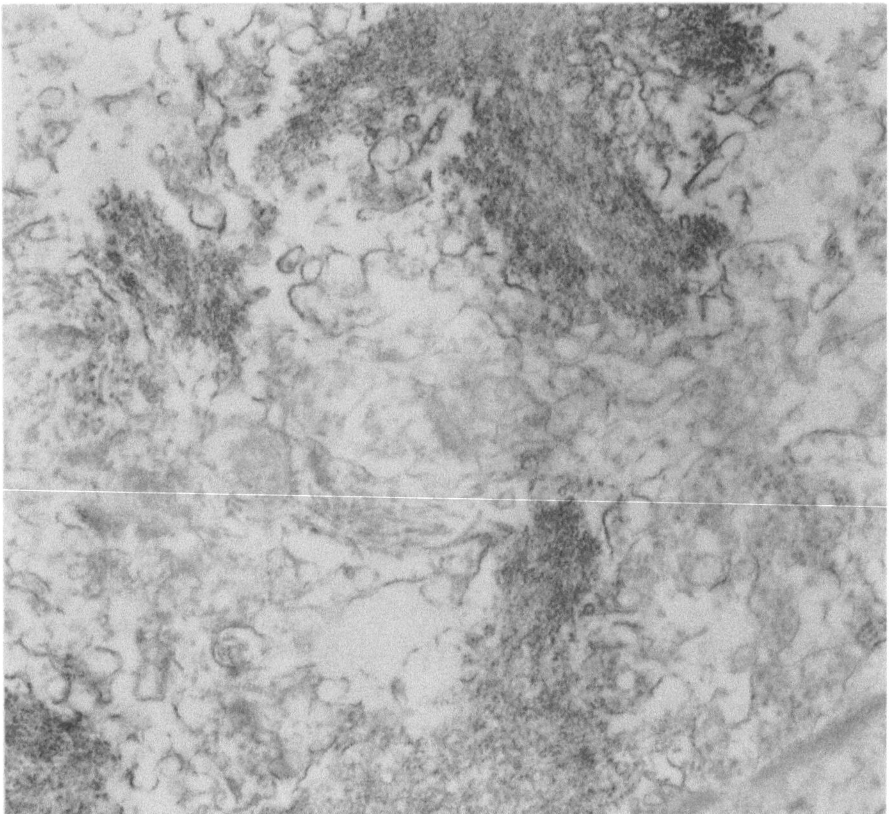

Fig. 4. Immunoelectron micrograph of the amyloid fibrils in senile plaques which were decorated by a positive DAB reaction product with an anti-C1q antibody. Other tissue elements such as neurofilaments, Alzheimer's neurofibrillary tangles, degenerated neuronal processes, or glial filaments were negative

like the neurites or the glia (Fig. 4). Sometimes only the peripheral parts of the amyloid plaques were stained. It is likely that this pattern indicates the difficulty with which the antibody penetrates into the tissue.

The presence of immunoglobulins and the complements C1q and C3 suggests that the amyloid in senile plaques is of an immune complex. We do not know what kind of substance or protein elicits the immunological reactions in the brain of patients with Alzheimer's disease, neither do we understand the operation of the autoimmune mechanism, or whether any infectious agent or agents are present. Powers et al. (1981) and Eikelenboom and Stam (1982) have speculated that the neurofilament protein might be involved. However, we have been unable to detect any neurofilament protein in the amyloid fibril of senile plaques (Ishii and Haga 1984). The findings of Powers et al. (1981) could have resulted from the use of contaminated antigens to raise the antibodies to neurofilaments.

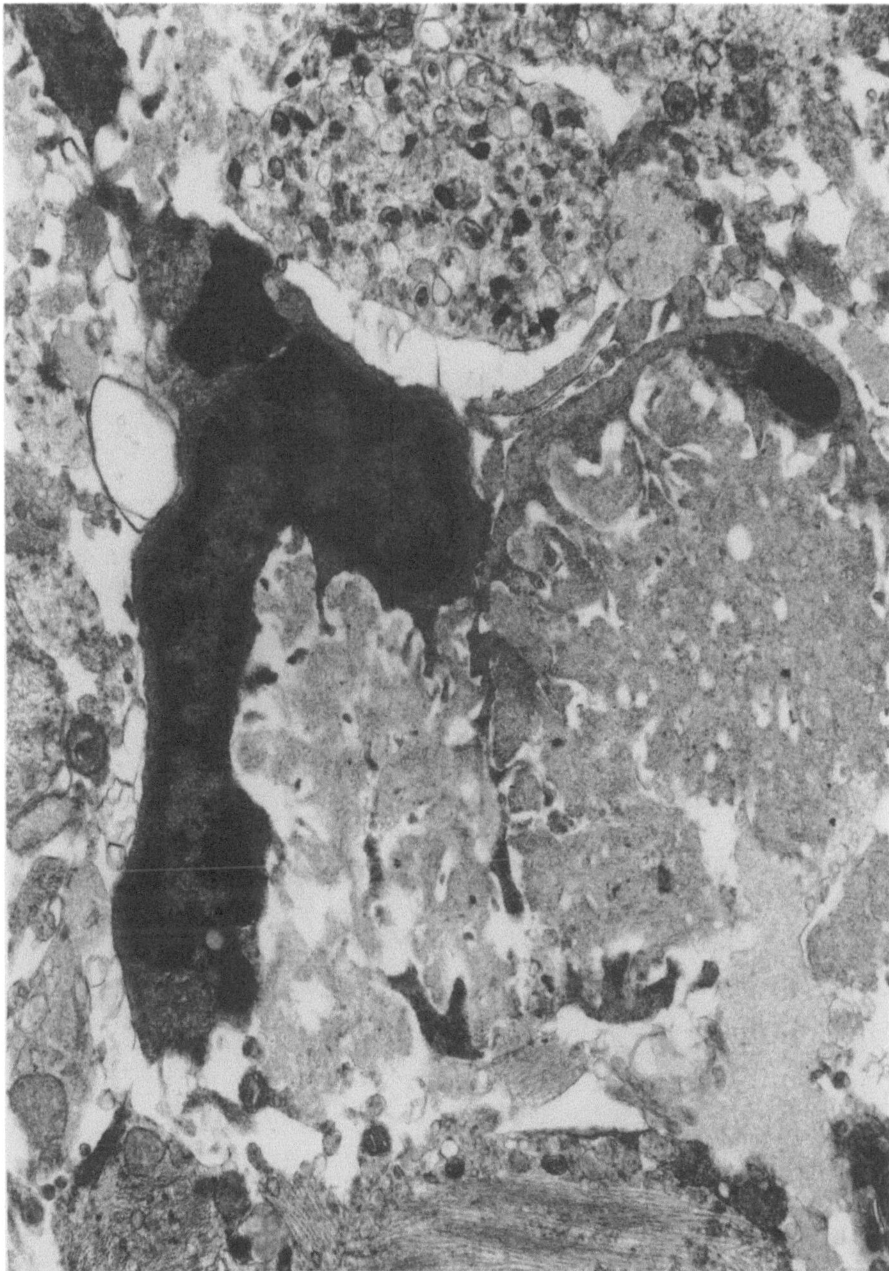

Fig. 5. Amyloid fibrils appeared to be produced near the cell membrane of a macrophage. Note the cell membrane has disappeared where amyloid fibrils seem to have emerged

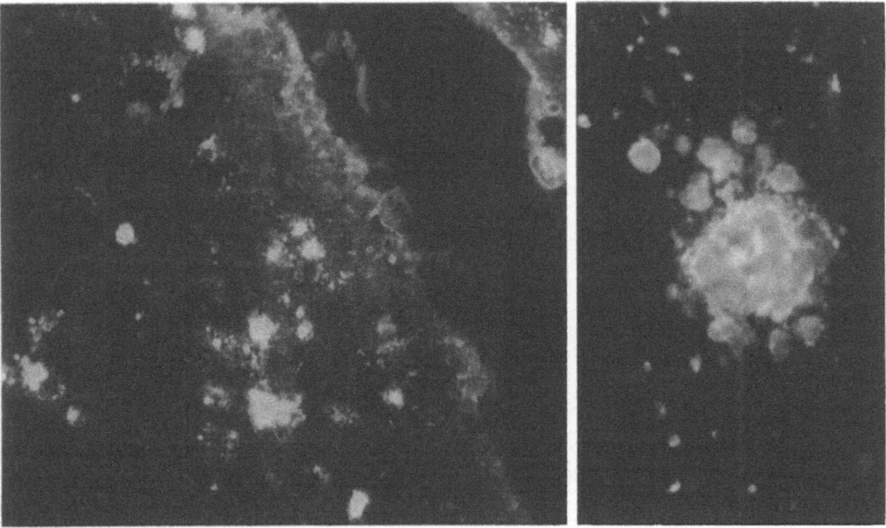

Fig. 6. Immunoblot of TEP fraction with complement C1q antibody. TEP fractions were prepared as described in "Materials and Methods" and aliquots of 3 µl were applied on micro 2 DE, before immunoblotting. *A:* TEP fraction from brain of a patient with Alzheimer's disease (KM, 84-year-old female), *B:* TEP fraction from the normal, aged brain

Fig. 7. Positive immunofluorescence of kuru plaques with anticomplement C1q antibody. *a* Many kuru plaques are positive in molecular layer of cerebellum. *b* Larger magnification of the positive kuru plaques, X 180

If the binding of C1q to the amyloid fibrils is immunological in nature, we do not know the mechanism by which the C1q was activated. The complement cascade can be activated in many ways by the immune complex, by fluid phase B (trypsin), by other substances such as the intermediate filaments (Linder et al. 1979), or by a C-reactive protein. However, we observed no reaction product of an HRP-anti-C1q binding on the intermediate filaments.

Shirahama et al. (1982) have claimed that prealbumin is the common constituent protein for both Alzheimer's tangles and the amyloid in senile plaques. However, no other reports have confirmed their findings. Complements C1q and C3 are also present in the amyloid plaques in the brain of patients with Creutzfeldt-Jakob disease (CJD) and Gerstman-Straussler-Scheinker disease (GSS) (Ishii et al. 1984, Fig. 7). In the amyloid plaques from brains of patients with CJD and GSS, complements C5 through C9 were also absent, showing an identical pattern of complement binding to that of the amyloid in senile plaques. A close relationship between unique proteins such as scrapie-associated fibrils (SAF) (Merz et al. 1981; Diringer et al. 1983) or prion (Prusiner 1982; Prusiner et al. 1983; Bockman et al. 1985) and amyloid plaques has been postulated (Merz et al. 1983, 1984; Prusiner et al. 1983). For instance, the morphology of these proteins is similar to that of amyloid (Merz et al. 1983; Prusiner et al. 1983), and the antibodies to a scrapie prion have reacted with the amyloid-like structure in the scrapie-infected hamster (Bendheim et al. 1984). Bockman et al. (1985) have maintained that amyloid plaques actually represent an aggregation of prions. Thus, direct involvement of an infectious agent in the amyloid deposition is suspected in this disease.

The antibody against the β-protein isolated by Glenner and Wong (1984) has been seen to react beautifully with the amyloid in senile plaques from the brain of patients with Alzheimer's disease and Down's syndrome. This protein has no homology with a known protein (Glenner and Wong 1984) and we do not yet know whether the β-protein of Glenner and Wong (1984) has an antigenic or an amyloidogenic property in Alzheimer's disease, similar to the abnormal prealbumin which constitutes the amyloidogenic polypeptide in familial amyloid neuropathy.

Our immunohistochemical study to find viral antigens in the brain of Alzheimer patients was unsuccessful (Ishii and Haga 1983a). We used a wide variety of antibodies to viruses, but were unable to find any antigens in the amyloid in senile plaques or in other tissue elements, though we did find, in one case, a fluorescence toward a JS virus (papova) in oligodendroglial cells. Likewise, estimations of the antibody titers toward a variety of neurotropic viruses in the blood and cerebrospinal fluid of patients with Alzheimer's disease have not produced any definite results (Ishii et al. 1982).

If the presence of C1q and C3 in the amyloid of senile plaques is an immune reaction triggered by an immune complex, this can explain the tissue damage surrounding the amyloid fibrils, i. e., the senile plaque formation. Complement binding, especially C3 binding, to the immune complex stimulates macrophages and accelerates their secretion of hydrolases (Shorlemmer et al. 1977). This kind of macrophage activity would induce damage and degeneration to the membranes of the neuronal processes. This interpretation supports our ultrastructural study of senile plaques which has shown that the most degenerated neuronal processes were reactive or secondary in nature (Ishii and Haga 1976b).

Acknowledgments. This study was supported by a grant-in-aid for general scientific research from the Ministry of Education, Science and Culture, grant No. 870303 from the National Center for Nervous, Mental, and Muscular Disorders (NCNMMD), and a grant for primary amyloidosis research from the Ministry of Health and Welfare, Japan.

References

Alafuzoff I, Adolfsson R, Grundke-Iqbal I, Winblad B (1987) Blood-brain barrier in Alzheimer dementia and in non-demented elderly. Acta Neuropathol (Berl) 73: 160–166

Alzheimer A (1907) Über eine eigenartige Erkrankung der Hirnrinde. Allg Z Psychiatr 64: 146–156

Bendheim PE, Barry RA, Dearmond SJ, Stites DP, Prusiner SB (1984) Antibodies to a scrapie prion protein. Nature 310: 418–421

Blessed G, Tomlinson BE, Roth M (1968) The association between quantitative measures of dementia and of senile change in the cerebral grey matter of elderly subjects. Br J Psychiatry 114: 797–811

Bockman JM, Kingsbury DT, McKinley MP, Bendheim PE, Prusiner SB (1985) Creutzfeldt-Jakob disease prion proteins in human brains. N Engl J Med 312: 73–78

Diringer H, Gelderblom H, Hilmert H, Ozel M, Edelbluth C (1983) Scrapie infectivity, fibrils and low molecular weight protein. Nature 306: 476–478

Eikelenboom P, Stam FC (1982) Immunoglobulins and complement factors in senile plaques. Acta Neuropathol (Berl) 57: 239–242

Glenner GG, Wong CW (1984) Alzheimer's disease: initial report of the purification and characterization of a novel cerebrovascular amyloid protein. Biochem Biophys Res Commun 120: 885–890

Goldgaber D, Lerman MI, McBride OW, Saffiotti U, Gajdusek DC (1987) Characterization and chromosomal localization of a cDNA encoding brain amyloid of Alzheimer's disease. Science 235: 877–880

Haga S, Shinoda T, Kato K, Aizawa T, Sato M, Saito T, Ishii T (1986) Association of senile plaques and microglia – a study with a monoclonal anti-macrophage antibody. Abstract of the 27th annual meeting of Japanese Neuropathological Society, p 131

Ihara Y, Kurizaki H, Nukina N, Sugita H, Toyokura Y, Ebara C (1981) Presence of immunoglobulin light chain in the cores of senile plaques – an unlabelled antibody peroxidase-antiperoxidase (PA) study. Neurol Med (Japan) 15: 292–295

Ishii T, Haga S (1976a) Immuno-electron microscopic localization of immunoglobulins in amyloid fibrils of senile plaques. Acta Neuropathol (Berl) 36: 243–249

Ishii T, Haga S (1976b) On the various forms of neurite and synapse degeneration. Recent Adv Res Nerv Syst (Japan) 20: 372–378

Ishii T, Haga S (1983a) Viral antigens in senile plaques. An immunofluorescent study. In: Hiraro A, Miyoshi K (eds) Proceedings of AINO Foundation symposium on the neuropsychiatric disorders of the aged. Tokyo, Igakushoin, pp 32–38

Ishii T, Haga S (1983b) The presence of immunoglobulins and complements in senile plaques – an immunofluorescent study. Neuropathology (Japan) 4: 31–36

Ishii T, Haga S (1984) Immuno-electron microscopic localization of complements in amyloid fibrils of senile plaques. Acta Neuropathol (Berl) 63: 296–300

Ishii T, Haga S, Shimizu F (1975) Identification of components of immunoglobulins in senile plaques by means of fluorescent antibody technique. Acta Neuropathol (Berl) 32: 157–162

Ishii T, Haga S, Oyanagi S, Tazima M, Kato K, Miyamura T (1982) Virus antibodies in the sera and cerebrospinal fluid (CSF) of patients with Alzheimer's disease and senile dementia (AHD-SD). In: Ohashi H, Nakayama K, Saito M, Saletu B (eds) Proceedings of World Psychiatric Association regional symposium. Kyoto, Japan, pp 261–264

Ishii T, Haga S, Yagishita S, Tateishi J (1984) The presence of complements in amyloid plaques of patients with Creutzfeldt-Jakob disease and Gerstman-Straussler-Scheiker disease. Appl Pathol 2: 370–379

Kang J, Lemaire HG, Unterback A, Salbaum JM, Masters CL, Grzeschik KH, Multhaup G, Beyreuther K, Muller-Hill B (1987) The precursor of Alzheimer's disease amyloid A4 protein resembles a cell-surface receptor. Nature 325: 733–736

Laemmli UK (1970) Cleavage of structural protein during head assembly of bacteriophage T4. Nature 227: 680–685

Linder E, Lehto VP, Stenman S (1979) Activation of complement by cytoskeletal intermediate filaments. Nature 278: 176–178

Masters CL, Simms G, Weiman NA, Multhaup G, McDonald BL, Beyreuther K (1985) Amyloid plaque core protein in Alzheimer disease and Down syndrome. Proc Nat Acad Sci USA 82: 4245–4249

Merz PA, Somerville RA, Wisniewski HM, Iqbal K (1981) Abnormal fibrils from scrapie-infected brain. Acta Neuropathol (Berl) 54: 63–74

Merz PA, Somerville RA, Wisniewski HM, Manuelidis I, Manuelidis EE (1983) Scrapie-associated fibrils in Creutzfeldt-Jakob disease. Nature 306: 474–476

Merz PA, Rohwer RG, Kascsak R, Wisniewski HM, Somerville RA, Gibbs CJ, Gajdusek DC (1984) Infection-specific particles from the unconventional slow virus diseases. Science 225: 437–440

Powers JM, Schlaepfer WW, Willingham MC, Hall BJ (1981) An immunoperoxidase study of senile cerebral amyloidosis with pathogenetic considerations. J Neuropathol Exp Neurol 40: 592–612

Prusiner SB (1982) Novel proteinaceous infectious particles cause scrapie. Science 216: 136–144

Prusiner SB, McKinley MP, Bowman KA, Bolton DC, Bendheim PE, Grothe DF, Glenner GG (1983) Scrapie prions aggregate to form amyloid-like birefringent rods. Cell 35: 349–358

Robakis NK, Wisniewski HM, Jenkins EC, Devin-Gage EA, Houck GE, Yao XL, Ramakrishna N, Wolfe G, Silverman WP, Brown WT (1987) Chromosome 21q21 sublocalisation of gene encoding beta-amyloid peptide in cerebral vessels and neuritic (senile) plaques of people with Alzheimer disease and Down syndrome. Lancet 1: 384–385

Schorlemmer HU, Ferluga J, Allison AC (1977) Interaction of macrophages and complement components in the pathogenesis of chronic inflammation. In: Willoughby D, Giroud JP, Velo GP (eds) Perspectives in inflammation. MTP Press, Lancaster, pp 191–206

Shirahama T, Skinner M, Westermark P, Rubinow A, Cohen AS, Brun S, Kemper TL (1982) Senile cerebral amyloid prealbumin as a common constituent in the neuritic plaque, in the neurofibrillary tangle, and in the microangiopathic lesion. Am J Pathol 107: 41–45

St George-Hyslop PH, Tanzi RE, Polinsky RJ, Haines JL, Nee L, Watkins PC, Myers RH, Feldman RG, Pollen D, Drachman D, Growdon J, Bruni A, Foncin J-F, Salmon D, Frommelt P, Amaducci L, Sorbi S, Piacentini S, Stewart GD, Hobb WY, Conneally PM, Gusella JF (1987) The genetic defect causing familial Alzheimer's disease maps on chromosome 21. Science 235: 885–890

Tanzi RE, Gusella JF, Watkins PC, Bruns GAP, St George-Hyslop P, Van Keuren MLV, Patterson D, Pagan S, Kurnit DM, Neve RL (1987) Amyloid β protein gene: cDNA, mRNA distribution, and genetic linkage near the Alzheimer locus. Science 235: 880–884

Towbin H, Staehelin T, Gordon J (1979) Electrophoretic transfer of proteins from polyacrylamide gels to nitrocellulose sheet: procedure and some applications. Proc Nat Acad Sci USA 76: 4350–4354

Wisniewski HM, Kozlowski P (1982) Evidence for blood-brain barrier changes in senile dementia of the Alzheimer type (SDAT) Ann NY Acad Sci 396: 119–129

The Blood-Brain Barrier in Cerebral Amyloidogenesis in Alzheimer's Disease and Scrapie

P. Eikelenboom, H. Fraser, J. M. Rozemuller, and *F. C. Stam*

Summary

There is a diversity of opinions concerning the defect in the blood-brain barrier permeability in Alzheimer's disease and in scrapie. In this paper we review the evidence for blood-brain barrier dysfunction and for serum factors and blood-borne cells in cerebral amyloidogenesis in Alzheimer's dementia and in scrapie. The hypothetical role of immunologically mediated injury to the central nervous system in both disorders is discussed. The basis of the different conclusions is identified, and much of the evidence supporting a systematic or haematogeneous origin for cerebral amyloidosis is shown to arise from the unreliability or variation in histochemical techniques, from the inappropriate use of "markers" and from false interpretations based on localisation of proteins and antigens. It is concluded that the primary pathogenesis of plaques occurs within the neuroparenchyma and that the evidence for systemic involvement remains inconclusive.

Introduction

Cerebral amyloid deposition is one of the major neuropathological changes in Alzheimer's dementia and aging. Senile cerebral amyloidosis occurs in senile plaques and in the walls of leptomeningeal and cortical arteries and arterioles. Amyloid plaques in experimental mouse scrapie are analogous in structure to senile plaques in Alzheimer's disease, although the major plaque core proteins differ between the two diseases. In Alzheimer's disease the main protein in both senile plaques and congophilic vessels is a 4-kd protein, A_4 or β-amyloid protein (Glenner and Wong 1984; Masters et al. 1985). In scrapie the protein cross-reacts antigenetically with the glycoprotein PrP (De Armond et al. 1985). There has been much progress in the characterization of cerebral amyloid fibrils in recent years, but information about the involvement of microenvironmental factors in amyloid formation is sparse. A role for extracerebral factors has been suggested by several authors. The involvement of these factors might result from a blood-brain barrier dysfunction with leakage of serum proteins into the neuropil (Wisniewski and Kozlowski 1982; Mann 1985; Hardy et al. 1986). The following mechanisms for the role of serum proteins in cerebral amyloid formation have been proposed:
1. Chronic "flooding" of the neuronal elements with serum proteins would "affect the performance of neuronal cells" (Wisniewski and Kozlowski 1982).

2. Neurotoxic factors of serum origin (such as immune complexes) may enter the brain due to primary blood-brain barrier dysfunction, leading to neuritic degeneration (Ishii et al. 1975; Ishii and Haga 1976; Hardy et al. 1986).
3. An intracerebral exudation of an abnormal precursor protein would lead to amyloid fibril deposition (Glenner 1979, 1986).

During amyloidogenesis, phagocytic cells are involved in amyloid deposition (Glenner 1980), and in cerebral amyloid these cells are described as either microglia or macrophages. Although the origin of these cells remains unresolved, it has been suggested that they are bone-marrow derived cells (Hikita et al 1985; Merz et al. 1987).

In this paper we review the evidence for blood-brain barrier dysfunction as well as for serum factors and blood-borne cells in cerebral amyloidogenesis in both Alzheimer's dementia and scrapie. In particular, the hypothetical role of immunologically mediated injury to the central nervous system in both disorders is discussed. It is concluded from the weight of evidence that the pathogenesis of plaques occurs within the neuroparenchyma and that the evidence for systemic involvement remains inconclusive.

Serum and Cerebrospinal Fluid

The evidence concerning immunoglobulin levels in patients with dementia states is conflicting. An inverse relationship between serum IgG concentration and measures of intelligence in elderly persons was found by Roseman and Buckley (1975). Cohen and Eisdorfer (1980) found significantly elevated IgG and IgA levels in cognitively impaired elderly persons, and serum IgG emerged as the best predictor of the test performance in such patients. Henschke et al. (1979) found higher mean serum levels of IgG only in patients with late-onset dementia. On the other hand, in presenile Alzheimer's dementia, Tavolato and Argentiero (1980) found a decrease in serum IgM levels but did not find elevated serum IgG levels. Again, in more recent studies, mean serum concentrations of IgG, IgM, IgA, IgE and IgD were not found to be different in patients with Alzheimer's dementia from those of control subjects (Jonker et al. 1982; Alafuzoff et al. 1983.

Cerebrospinal fluid (CSF) studies have been performed to provide information regarding both the integrity of the blood-brain barrier and antibody production within the CNS. The level of CSF immunoglobulins is influenced both by the concentration of the serum globulins and by the permeability of the blood-brain barrier. This can be misleading unless the measurements of the concentrations of immunoglobulins and albumin both in the serum and in the CSF are taken into account. Under normal conditions a linear relationship is found between the CSF/serum ratio of albumin. Increased immunoglobulin concentration in the CSF due to production within the CNS shows a deviation from such a relationship. For IgG, IgM, IgA and IgD such a deviation was not found in patients with Alzheimer's dementia (Jonker et al. 1982). In electrophoretic analysis of CSF, Williams et al. (1980) found oligoclonal bands in the gamma globulin region in five out of eight patients with a clinical diagnosis of presenile Alzheimer's dementia. We did not observe multiple banding within the gamma globulin fraction of CSF in patients with Alzheimer's dementia (Jonker et al. 1982). The conclusion that there is no synthesis of immunoglobulins within the CNS in Alzheimer's dementia is in agreement with recent CSF studies (Alafuzoff et al. 1983; Chapel et al. 1984; Elovaara et al. 1985; Kay et al. 1987). An increased CSF/serum ratio for albumin suggesting an increased blood-brain barrier permeability has been reported by Alafuzoff et al. (1985) and Elovaara et al. (1985) but could not be confirmed by other investigators (Leonardi et al. 1985; Kay et al. 1987)

In sheep with natural or experimentally induced scrapie, Collis et al. (1979) found that the concentration of IgG in serum was increased in a high proportion of sheep in the clinical stage of the disease. Further studies showed that the increased concentrations of IgG in CSF are due to passive filtration from serum and not to local antibody production in the CNS (Collis and Kimberlin 1983).

Cerebral Amyloidosis and Plasma proteins

With immunofluorescence, Stam (1965) demonstrated immunoglobulins in senile plaques. Later Ishii and co-workers (Ishii et al. 1975; Ishii and Haga 1976) and Torack and Lynch (1981) reported the presence of immunoglobulins in senile plaques and in congophilic angiopathy. These authors suggested that brain amyloid fibrils are derived from immunoglobulins. Immunohistoperoxidase studies carried out on formolfixed paraffin sections showed that the amyloid depositions in senile plaques and vascular vessels exhibited a positive reaction for IgG, IgG (Fc-specific), IgM, IgA, kappa and lambda light chains, fibrinogen, albumins and other plasma proteins (Powers et al. 1981; Mann et al. 1982). These authors suggest that the positive immunohistochemical reactions demonstrated within senile plaques and congophilic angiopathy are more likely to result from leakage of plasma proteins, including immunoglobulins, than to indicate the involvement of immunological mechanisms in the aetiology of plaques. This supports the opinion of Katenkamp et al. (1970) that the presence of IgG in senile plaques is due to exudation of plasma proteins.

Using immunohistoperoxidase techniques we have studied the presence of plasma proteins in senile plaques and congophilic angiopathy both on brief acetone-fixed cryostat sections and on formol-fixed paraffin sections (Eikelenboom and Stam 1982, 1984; Stam and Eikelenboom 1985; Rozemuller et al. submitted). The immunohistoperoxidase findings on acetone-fixed cryostat sections are summarized in Table 1. With antisera against IgG, we observed a weak peroxidase activity in the corona of some plaques and no activity in the amyloid core. A similar staining pattern was found with antisera against IgG (γ-specific) and IgG (Fc-specific). No plaques reacted with antisera against IgM (μ-specific), IgA (α-specific), fibrinogen, albumin and ceruloplasmin. Using antisera against the different complement factors, we found on cryostat sections that all senile plaques, especially the amyloid cores, contain C1q, C4 and C3. We could not demonstrate C5, C3 pro-activator, properdin or C-reactive protein in senile plaques. When the immunohistoperoxidase staining for immunoglobulins, fibrinogen and albumin was followed by Congo red staining, we found that congophilic arteries and capillaries showed sporadic peroxidase activity at the sites of vascular amyloid deposits. Peroxidase activity was evident in the endothelial layer and especially in the adventitia of the blood vessels. Few peroxidase-positive amyloid

Table 1. Immunohistoperoxidase detection of plasma proteins in acetone-fixed cryostat sections in Alzheimer's disease

Antisera against plasma proteins	Vascular amyloid	Senile plaque Corona	Amyloid core
IgG(γ-specific)	(−)	(+)	−
IgA(α-specific)	(−)	−	−
IgM (μ-specific)	(−)	−	−
Lambda chains	(−)	(−)	−
Kappa chains	(−)	(−)	−
Albumin	(−)	−	−
Fibrinogen	(−)	−	−
Prealbumin	−	−	−
C1q	(+)	+	++
C3c	(+)	+	++
C5	(−)	−	−
Properdin	(−)	−	−
C3 proactivator	(−)	−	−
P component	(+)	(−)	(−)
A component	−	−	−

Symbols: −, no labelling; (−), occasional labelling; (+), labelling of most deposits; +, consistent labelling; ++, strong labelling

deposits were detected in medium-sized congophilic cerebral arteries with antisera against fibrinogen, albumin and immunoglobulins, especially IgG. With antisera against C1q, C4 and C3 more vascular amyloid depositions were stained than with antisera against other plasma proteins, but some unstained congophilic vessels were also seen.

Using immunohistoperoxidase techniques on formol-fixed paraffin sections, Shirahama et al. (1982) found prealbumin associated with senile plaques and congophilic microangiopathy. In contrast to their findings, we could not detect prealbumin in amyloid plaques and congophilic angiopathy neither on acetone-fixed cryostat sections nor on formol-fixed paraffin sections. Our results of immunohistoperoxidase staining for plasma proteins on formol-fixed paraffin sections compared with on acetone-fixed cryostat sections are summarised in Table 2. In paraffin sections, amyloid cores of senile plaques were occasionally stained for IgG, complement factors C1q and C3, albumin and fibrinogen. Except for complement factors, the intensity of peroxidase staining of senile plaques correlated strongly with diffuse staining of the parenchyma around senile plaques. Alafuzoff et al. (1987) reported that, on formol-fixed paraffin sections, no staining of plaques above background was observed with antialbumin and antifibrinogen. In our opinion the conflicting reports about the presence of plasma proteins in senile plaques on formol-fixed paraffin sections can be explained by a great internal variability, by background staining, and by negative effects of the formol fixation and paraffin embedding on the presence of complement factors (Stam and Eikelenboom 1985; Rozemuler et al. submitted).

In IM mice affected by scrapie following intracerebral infection with the high-plaque agent 81V (incubation period 300–320 days), immunohistoperoxidase stain-

Table 2. Immunohistoperoxidase detection of plasma proteins in acetone-fixed cryostat sections and 1-week formol-fixed paraffin sections in Alzheimer's disease

Antisera against	Acetone-fixed cryostat sections			Formol-fixed paraffin sections		
	Paren-chymal cells	Plaque amyloid	Blood vessels	Paren-chymal cells	Plaque amyloid	Blood vessels
IgG	− or (+)	−	+	− or ++	− or (+)	− or (+)
Albumin	− or (+)	−	+	− or ++	− or (+)	− or (+)
Fibrinogen	− or (+)	−	+	− or (+)	− or (+)	− or (+)
Prealbumin	−	−	−	−	−	−
C1q	−	++	(+)	−	− or (+)	−
C3c	−	++	(+)	−	− or (+)	−

Symbols: −, no labelling; (+), labelling in some cells, plaques or blood vessels; +, many cells, plaques or blood vessels are positively labelled; ++, large field with labelled cells, all amyloid plaques are labelled; − or (+), − or ++, considerable variations in staining in and between the cases

ing did not detect albumin, fibrinogen, immunoglobulins or complement factors C1q and C3 in amyloid plaques. In amyloid plaques of autolytic brains, no peroxidase activity was found after staining for C1q and C3 (Eikelenboom et al. 1987).

Blood-Brain Barrier

There is only indirect evidence for increased permeability of cortical vasculature in Alzheimer's dementia based on the extravasation of plasma proteins into the brain parenchyma. With immunocytochemical techniques plasma proteins have been described in amyloid plaques, congophilic angiopathy, and in neuronal cells and astrocytes. Wisniewski and Kozlowski (1982) found that neuronal and glial cells and plaques were heavily stained with both anti-albumin and anti-globulin, especially in those areas of the cortex where the plaques were numerous. In addition they reported that all plaques were surrounded with reactive astrocytes which were also heavily stained with both antisera. In our work we did not observe an association between areas of IgG and albumin containing neuronal cells and astrocytes with high numbers of senile plaques. Sometimes large numbers of neuronal cells and astrocytes staining for plasma proteins were seen in areas with only a few amyloid plaques, while areas with numerous senile plaques remained unstained. There was no indication from microscopic observation that congophilic angiopathy was more frequently associated with clusters of neuronal cells and astrocytes positively stained for plasma proteins than could be expected in a random distribution (Rozemuller et al., submitted). We also compared the occurrence of extravascular plasma proteins in the brain parenchyma of patients with Alzheimer's dementia with that in age-matched, non-demented controls, with and without other neuropathological disorders. Cases in the group with Alzheimer's dementia and both control groups included ones with large fields of neuronal cells and astrocytes, positively stained for IgG and albumin. These clusters of positively stained neurons and astrocytes were found in 15 of 28 cases with Alzheimer's dementia, 7 of 13 non-demented cases with other neuropathological disorders and 4 of 18 cases without neuropathological disorders. In three cases of Alzheimer's dementia we could not stain neuronal cells or astrocytes for albumin or IgG and in ten cases only a few neurons and astrocytes stained. In formol-fixed brains obtained at post mortem Esiri et al. (1976) noted a widespread binding of immunoglobulins and other plasma proteins to neurons, glia and other CNS constituents, both in a number of neuropathological conditions and in patients who died suddenly without evidence of CNS disease. These observations of Esiri and co-workers and our own findings led us to conclude that the cytochemical detection of plasma proteins in the neuropil cannot be used as evidence of a blood-brain barrier defect in Alzheimer's dementia or any other neurological disease.

In scrapie, Wisniewski et al. (1983) showed focal extravasation of intravenously injected horseradish peroxidase (HRP) in terminally affected mice. Recently we studied the permeability of the blood-brain barrier at intervals throughout the incubation period of the same scrapie model (87V agent in IM mice) using the immunocytochemical demonstration of plasma proteins and by intravenous injection of HRP (Eikelenboom et al. 1987). Using immunohistoperoxidase techniques for fibrinogen, immunoglobulin and complement factors, staining was confined to the lumen of blood vessels and no staining was found in the neuropil, in neuronal cells or in astrocytes. For albumin, immunohistoperoxidase staining showed a weak positive reaction in the neuropil around almost all blood vessels in both normal and scrapie-affected mice but no staining was found in neuronal cells and astrocytes. After intravenously injecting HRP there was no abnormal leakage of HRP either around cerebral vessels or amyloid plaques. Our findings suggest that there is little or no leakage of plasma proteins into the brain parenchyma in preclinical and scrapie-affected mice and that the blood-brain barrier is therefore essentially intact.

Microglia

It is generally accepted that phagocytic cells are essential for the deposition of amyloid by proteolytic cleavage of amyloidogenic precursor proteins (Glenner 1980). There are several studies suggesting that, in both Alzheimer's dementia and scrapie, phagocytic cells described either as microglia or marcophages are involved in amyloid plaque formation (Wisniewski and Terry 1973; Bruce and Fraser 1975; Wisniewski et al. 1981; Wisniewski and Merz 1983; Moretz et al. 1983; Hikita et al. 1985). Using enzyme histochemical and immunohistochemical methods we have recently investigated the nature of the cells around amyloid plaques in Alzheimer's dementia and scrapie (Rozemuller et al. 1986; Ekelenboom et al. 1987). Acid phosphatase and non-specific esterase are used as a non-specific enzyme histochemical marker for macrophages. Around different types of senile plaques, no increase of acid-phosphatase-positive cells was found in comparison with the rest of the grey matter. Acid phosphatase activity was always present in the corona of senile plaques but staining was too strong to permit the identification of individual cells. Friede (1965) and Krigman et al. (1965) have described an increase in acid phosphatase-positive cells in the cerebral cortex of patients with Alzheimer's dementia.

Table 3. Antibody panel for macrophages in humans

Antibody	Cluster of designation (CD)	Predominant specificity
DakoLC (DLC)	CD45	Leucocyte lineage
OKIa	–	HLA-DR (class II MHC)
α1-Antichymotrypsin	–	Monohistiocytic cell series
Lysozyme	–	Myeloid cells, monocytes Reactive histiocytes
Mo-1	CD11^B	Complement receptor 3
OKM 1	CD11^B	Complement receptor 3
OKM 5	–	Monocytes, platelets
C3brec	CD35	B cells, monocytes, Granulocyte cells,
FK24	CD11^c	Myeloid cells, monocytes Macrophages (p150/95)
LeuM5	CD11^c	Monocytes/macrophages (p150/95)
LeuM3	CD14	Monocytes/macrophages
Leu 11^b	CD16	Low-affinity Fc receptor
MY4	CD14	Mononuclear-phagocytic lineage
EBM 11		Mononuclear-phagocytic lineage
5D2		Low-avidity Fc receptor

For references to the antibody panel, see Rozemuller et al. (1986)

Our findings do not confirm a relationship between acid phosphatase-positive cells and senile plaques (Rozemuller et al. 1986). Non-specific esterase was observed in neurons and sporadically in a few cells (probably small neurons) located in the corona of some plaques. Using a panel of antibodies with specificities predominantly for mononuclear phagocytes (see Table 3), cells were characterised in and around senile plaques. The results are summarised in Table 4. With antibodies EBM/11 and MY4

Table 4. Immunohistoperoxidase findings with macrophage markers in Alzheimer's disease

Antisera	Amyloid plaques	Congophilic angiopathy	Small glial cells subcortical	Small glial cells grey matter
DLC	–	–	–	–
OKIa	–/+	–	+	(+)
α-1-Antichymotrypsin	–/+	–	(+)	(+)
Lysozyme	–	–	–	–
Mo-1	–	–	–	–
OKM1	–	–	–	–
OKM5	–	–	–	–
α-C3brec	–	–	–	–
FK24	–/+	–	(+)	–
Leu M5	–/+	–	+	(+)
Leu M3	–	–	–	–
Leu 11b	–	–	–	–
MY4	+/–	–	+	(+)
EBM/11	+/–	–	(+)	(+)
5D2	–	–	–	–

Symbols: –, no labelling; –/+, some amyloid plaques are labelled; +/–, most amyloid plaques labelled; (+), some labelled cells dispersed in the cerebral cortex outside the senile plaques; +, cells are labelled

Table 5. Haemopoietic cell markers in mice

Monoclonal	Directed against
M 1/70 (Mac-1)	Complement receptor C3
ER-TR3	Antigens encoded in the Ia region of the H2 complex
NLDC-145	Non-lymphoid dendritic cells

For references, see Eikelenboom et al. (1987)

there was positive labelling of cells, although in some senile plaques no labelling occurred. With EBM/11, staining occurred in the cytoplasm, whereas with MY4, the cell membranes of small-branched glial cells were stained. The EBM/11- and MY4-positive cells were negative for the astrocyte marker GFAP. After staining with OKIa and FK24, cell processes of small glial cells were positive in some plaques. With the monoclonals EBM/11, MY4, OKIa and FK24, a few cortical and many subcortical glial cells were positively labelled. Using an α-1 antichymotrypsin antibody, there was a weak diffuse staining of the corona of some senile plaques and also a weak staining of some neuronal and glial cells dispersed in the grey and the white matter. The reactivity for α-1-antichymotrypsin resembled the staining for serum proteins. With a lot of well-known macrophage markers (e. g. LCA, Mo-1, α-C3brec, Leu M3, a-lysozyme), no labelled cells were found in or around senile plaques. With the antisera listed in Table 3 we did not observe labelled cells associated with the amyloid deposits in congophilic vessels.

In 87V scrapie-affected IM mice, cells associated with the amyloid plaques in the cerebral cortex did not show acid phosphatase activity, and there was only sporadically a weak non-specific esterase activity. The haemopoietic cell markers used for cell identity are listed in Table 5. In scrapie-affected brains, only a few cells in the white matter stained faintly for Mac-1. Amyloid plaques sometimes showed a weak diffuse positive staining for Mac-1. However, with Mac-1, as well as with the monoclonals ER-TR3 and NLDC-145, no labelled cells were found to be associated with the plaques. With antisera against the astrocyte marker GFAP, positive cells were located in clusters and amyloid plaques were always found with a close spatial relationship to these clusters. It can be concluded, therefore, that there is no evidence that blood-borne monocytes are involved in the local microenvironment of cerebral amyloidogenesis.

Discussion

Involvement of plasma factors from blood-brain barrier dysfunction in amyloid plaque formation has been suggested by several authors (Ishii et al. 1975; Ishii and Haga 1976; Glenner 1979, 1986; Wisniewski and Kozlowski 1982). However, apart from some complement factors, plasma proteins are not found consistently in congophilic arteries or in amyloid plaques. It has been assumed that the immunostaining of plaques for IgG and complement factors is due to the presence of antigen/antibody complexes in amyloid plaques (Ishii et al. 1975; Ishii and Haga 1976, 1984; Pouplard and Emile 1985; Alafuzoff et al. 1987). However, on acetone-fixed cryostat sections, positive staining for immunoglobulins was seen in the corona of only some plaques and was never observed in the amyloid core. On formol-fixed paraffin sections, the amyloid cores occasionally contained plasma proteins but, apart from complement factors, the staining of senile plaques for the other plasma proteins was related to the background staining. In congophilic arteries most amyloid deposits were positive for complement factors but not for other plasma proteins including immunoglobulins.

These findings do not support the assumption that the presence of complement factors in senile plaques and congophilic angiopathy indicate the presence of antigen/antibody complexes. Investigations of serum and CSF also fail to support the hypothesis that cerebral amyloidosis is the result of an autoimmune response (Jonker et al. 1982; Stam et al., in press).

CSF studies of protein concentrations do not support the hypothesis of a diffuse disruption of the blood-brain barrier as a pathogenic mechanism in Alzheimer's dementia (Kay et al. 1987). In addition, a positron-emission tomographic study with rubidium 82 demonstrated normal impermeability for that ion in patients with Alzheimer's dementia (Friedland et al. 1983).

In brains obtained post mortem from both demented and non-demented patients, with or without other neuropathological disorders, there is a widespread binding of plasma proteins to various CNS constituents. Esiri et al. (1976) assumed that this binding was the result of a long post mortem delay, but Rozemuller et al. (submitted) found similar results in brains with a post mortem delay of only 2 h. Influences of agonal or post mortem changes on binding of plasma proteins to constituents of the neuropil cannot be ruled out. It is possible that these conditions concern especially damaged (degenerating) cells (Rozemuller et al. submitted). Positive immunohistoperoxidase staining for complement factors in the amyloid cores of senile plaques is a very consistent finding in cryostat sections. There are different explanations for the presence of complement factors in senile plaques. Firstly, there is a post mortem leakage of plasma proteins. The consistent finding of complement factors in senile plaques is not related to the presence of other plasma proteins and the possibility exists that complement factors bind selectively to amyloid fibres. We failed to detect complement factors in amyloid plaques from scrapie-affected mice, even if autolysis had been allowed to take place. Another explanation is that the complement factors are passed ante mortem from the blood into the neuropil, but as we discussed above there is no convincing evidence of a blood-brain barrier dysfunction with leakage of plasma proteins into the neuropil. A third explanation is that complement factors are produced by glial cells. Using clonal cells belonging to the astrocyte lineage, Mallat and Levi-Strauss (1987) have recently found that glial cells can produce the complement components C3 and factor B. Therefore, the presence of complement factors in senile plaques cannot be used as a priori evidence for a contribution from plasma in cerebral amyloidogenesis. In our opinion the cytochemical detection of plasma proteins in the neuropil cannot be considered as a reliable technique to investigate blood-brain barrier defects in neuropathological disorders (Rozemuller et al. submitted).

Reactive microglial cells may be involved in cerebral amyloid formation. The origin and function of microglial cells is still not resolved. According to Oehmichen (1982), microglia can be divided into resting and reactive types. Reactive microglial cells have strong cytoplasmic acid phosphatase and non-specific esterase activty and Fc- and

C3b-receptors on their membranes, whereas resting microglial cells are negative for these markers. It is suggested that reactive microglial cells, more appropriately called "brain macrophages", are only seen in damaged brains and are derived from blood-borne monocytes whilst resting microglial cells are of neuroectodermal origin. Cross-reactivity between leucocytes and brain cells is a well-known phenomenon (Budka and Majdic 1985; Merrill 1987). Positivity in glial cells for class II MHC antigens has been described by several authors. Functions carried out elsewhere by macrophages, such as antigen presentation and interleukin-1 production, can be performed in the brain by glial cells (Fontana et al. 1982; Fierz et al. 1985; Merrill 1987). These glial cells and macrophages appear to have similar functions and to share some character-istic proteins, enzymes and receptors. Although immunohistoperoxidase studies have shown that glial cells and macrophages share some epitopes, it would not be justified to conclude that these cells have common origin. With well-known macrophage markers, the glial cells associated with amyloid plaques are unlabelled. With all the macrophage markers we failed to find labelled cells associated with amyloid deposits in congophilic arteries (Rozemuller et al. 1987). In scrapie-affected mice we did not find cells belonging to the monocyte-macrophage lineage in association with amyloid plaques. Therefore, the weight of evidence, using macrophage markers, is that no cells belonging to the monocyte-macrophage lineage are involved in cerebral amyloid formation in either Alzheimer's dementia or scrapie.

In conclusion, there is no evidence for a blood-brain barrier dysfunction or for the involvement of plasma proteins or blood-borne cells in the cerebral amyloidogenesis in Alzheimer's disease or scrapie.

Acknowledgments. The work reviewed in this study was partly supported by grants from the stimulation fund for gerontology, SOOM, projects 840812 and 860812.

References

Alafuzoff I, Adolfsson R, Bucht G, Winbald B (1983) Albumin and immunoglobulin in plasma and cerebrospinal fluid and blood-cerebrospinal fluid barrier function in patients with dementia of Alzheimer's disease and multi-infarct dementia. J Neurol Sci 60: 465–472

Alafuzoff I, Adolfsson R, Grundke-Iqbal I, Winblad B (1985) Perivascular deposits of serum proteins in cerebral cortex in vascular dementia. Acta Neuropathol (Berl) 66: 292–298

Alafuzoff I, Adolfsson R, Grundke-Iqbal I, Winblad B (1987) Blood-brain barrier in Alzheimer dementia and in non-demented elderly. Acta Neuropathol (Berl) 73: 160–166

Bruce ME, Fraser H (1975) Amyloid plaques in the brains of mice infected with scrapie: morpho-logical variation and staining properties. Neuropathol Appl Neurobiol 1: 189–202

Budka H, Majdic O. (1985) Shared antigenic determinants between human hemopoietic cells and nervous tissues and tumors. Acta Neuropathol (Berl) 67: 58–66

Chapel HM, Esiri MM, Wilcock GK (1984) Immunoglobulin and other proteins in the cerebrospinal fluid of patients with Alzheimer's disease. J Clin Pathol 37: 697–699

Cohen D, Eisorfer C (1980) Serum immunoglobulins and cognitive status in the elderly: I. A population study. Br J Psychiatry 136: 33–39

Collis SC, Kimberlin RH (1983) Further studies on changes in immunoglobulin G in the sera and CSF of Herdwick sheep with natural and experimental scrapie. J Comp Pathol 93: 331–338

Collis SC, Kimberlin RH, Millson GC (1979) Immunoglobulin G concentration in the sera of Herdwick sheep with natural scrapie. J Comp Pathol 89: 389–396

DeArmond, SJ, McKinley MP, Barry RA, Branfeld MB, McColloch JR, Prusiner SB (1985) Identifi-cation of prion amyloid filament in scrapie-infected brain. Cell 41: 221–235

Eikelenboom, P, Stam FC (1982) Immunoglobulins and complement factors in senile plaques. An immunoperoxidase study. Acta Neuropathol (Berl) 57: 239–242

Eikelenboom P, Stam FC (1984) An immunohistochemical study on cerebral vascular and senile plaque amyloid in Alzheimer's. Virchows Arch [B] 47: 17–25

Eikelenboom P, Scott JR, McBride PA, Rozemuller JM, Bruce ME, Fraser H (1987) No evidence for involvement of plasmaproteins or blood-borne cells in amyloid plaque formation in scrapie-affected mice. Virchows Arch [B] 53: 251–256

Elovaara I, Icen A, Palo J, Erkinjuntti T (1985) CSF in Alzheimer's disease. Studies on blood-brain barrier function and intrathecal protein synthesis. J Neurol Sci 70: 73–80

Esiri MM, Taylor CR, Mason DY (1976) Application of an immunoperoxidase method to a study on the central nervous system: preliminary findings in a study on human formalin-fixed material. Neuropathol Appl Neurobiol 2: 233–246

Fierz W, Endler B, Reske K, Wekerle H, Fontana A (1985) Induction of Ia antigen expression on astrocytes by T cells. Gamma immune interferon and its effect on antigen presentation. J Immunol 134: 3785–3793

Fontana A, Kristensen F, Dubs R, Gemsa D, Weber E (1982) Production of prostaglandin E and an interleukin-1 like factor by cultured astrocytes and C6 glioma cells. J Immunol 129: 2413–2419

Friede RL (1965) Enzyme histochemical studies of senile plaques. J Neuropathol Exp Neurol 24: 477–491

Friedland RP, Yano Y, Budinger TF, Ganz E, Huesman RH, Derenzo SE, Knittel B (1983) Quantitative evaluation of blood brain barrier integrity in Alzheimer-type dementia: positron emission tomographic studies with rubidium-82. Eur Neurol (Suppl) 22: 19–20

Glenner GG (1979) Congophilic microangiopathy in the pathogenesis of Alzheimer's syndrome (presenile dementia). Med Hypotheses 5: 1231–1236

Glenner GG (1980) Amyloid deposits and amyloidosis. N Engl J Med 302: 1283–1291, 1333–1343

Glenner GG (1986) On primal causes in Alzheimer's disease. Neurobiol Aging 7: 506–508

Glenner GG, Wong CW Y(1984) Alzheimer's disease and Down's syndrome: sharing of a unique cerebrovascular amyloid fibril protein. Biochem Biophys Res Commun 122: 1131–1135

Hardy JA, Mann DMA, Wester P, Winblad B (1986) An integrative hypothesis concerning the pathogenesis and progression of Alzheimer's disease. Neurobiol Aging 7: 489–502

Henschke PJ, Bell DA, Cape RTD (1979) Immunologic indices in Alzheimer dementia. J Clin Exp Gerontol 1: 23–37

Hikita K, Tateishi J, Nagara H (1985) Morphogenesis of amyloid plaques in mice with Creutzfeldt-Jakob disease. Acta Neuropathol (Berl) 68: 138–144

Ishii T, Haga S, Schimuzu F (1975) Identification of components of immunoglobulins in senile plaques by means of fluorescent antibody technique. Acta Neuropathol (Berl) 32: 157–162

Ishii T, Haga S (1976) Immuno-electron microscopic localization of immunoglobulins in amyloid fibrils of senile plaques. Acta Neuropathol (Berl) 36: 243–249

Ishii T, Haga S (1984) Immuno-electron microscopic localization of complements in amyloid fibrils of senile plaques. Acta Neuropathol (Berl) 63: 296–300

Jonker C, Eikelenboom P, Tavenier P (1982) Immunological indices in the cerebrospinal fluid of patients with presenile dementia of the Alzheimer type. Br J Psychiatry 140: 44–49

Katenkamp D, Stiller D, Thoss K (1970) Untersuchungen zum immunohistochemischen Verhalten der senilen Plaques des menschlichen Gehirnes. Virchows Arch [A] 351: 333–339

Kay AD, May C, Papadopoulos NM, Costello R, Atack JR, Luxenberg JS, Cutler NR (1987) CSF and serum concentrations of albumin and IgG in Alzheimer's disease. Neurobiol Aging 8: 21–25

Krigman MR, Feldman RG, Bench K (1965) Alzheimer's presenile dementia – a histochemic and electronmicroscopic study. Lab Invest 14: 381–396

Leonardi A, Gaandolfo C, Caponnetto C, Arata L, Vecchia R (198) The integrity of the blood-brain barrier in Alzheimer's type and multi-infarct dementia evaluated by the study of albumin and IgG in the serum and cerebrospinal fluid. J Neurol Sci 67: 253–261

Mallat M, Levi-Strauss M (1987) Astrocytic production of complement components: C3c and factor B (Abstract). J Neuroimmunol 16: 114–115

Mann DMA (1985) The neuropathology of Alzheimer's disease: a review with pathogenetic, aetiological and therapeutic considerations. Mech Ageing Dev 31: 213–255

Mann DMA, Davies JS, Hawkes J, Yates PO (1982) Immunohistochemical staining of senile plaques. Neuropathol Appl Neurobiol 8: 55–61

Masters CL, Simms G, Weinman NA, Multhaup G, McDonald BL, Beyreuther K (1985) Amyloid plaque core protein in Alzheimer disease and Down syndrome. Proc Natl Acad Sci USA 82: 4245–4249

Merrill JE (1987) Macroglia: neural cells responsive to lymphokines and growth factors. Immunol Today 8: 146–150

Merz GS, Schwenk V, Schuller-Levis S, Gruca S, Wisniewski HM (1987) Isolation and characterization of macrophages from scrapie-infected mouse brain. Acta Neuropathol (Berl) 72: 240–247

Moretz RC, Wisniewski HM, Lossinski AS (1983) Pathogenesis of neuritic and amyloid plaques in scrapie – ultrastructural study of early changes in the cortical neuropil. In: Samuel D et al. (eds) Aging of the brain. Raven, New York, pp 61–79

Oehmichen M (1982) Are resting and/or reactive microglia macrophages? Immunobiology 161: 246–254

Pouplard A, Emile J (1985) New immunological findings in senile dementia. Interdisc Top Gerontol 19: 62–71

Powers JM, Schlaepfer WW, Willingham MC, Hall BJ (1981) An immunoperoxidase study of senile cerebral amyloidosis with pathogenetic considerations. J Neuropathol Exp Neurol 40: 592–612

Roseman JM, Buckley CE (1975) Inverse relationship between serum IgG concentration and measures of intelligence in elderly persons. Nature 254: 55–56

Rozemuller JM, Eikelenboom P, Stam FC (1986) Role of microglia in plaque formation in senile dementia of the Alzheimer type. An immunohistochemical study. Virchows Arch [B] 51:247–254

Rozemuller JM, Masters CL, Beyreuther K, Eikelenboom P, Stam FC (1987) Cerebral amyloidosis in Alzheimer's disease. Senile plaques and congophilic angiopathy (abstract). In: Pepeu G et al. (eds) New trends in aging research. Sirmione, Italy, p 96

Rozemuller JM, Eikelenboom P, Stam FC Blood-brain barrier dysfunction and Alzheimer's disease. (Submitted for publication)

Shirahama T, Skinner M, Westermark P, Rubinow A, Cohen AS, Brun A, Kemper TL (1982) Senile cerebral amyloid. Prealbumin as a common constituent in the neuritic plaque, in the neurofibrillary tangle, and in the microangiopathic lesion. Am J Pathol 107: 41–50

Stam FC (1965) Histochemistry of the senile involution of the brain. In: Luthy F, Bischoff A (eds) Proceedings of the fifth international congress of neuropathology. Excerpta Medica, Amsterdam, pp 513–517

Stam FC, Eikelenboom P (1985) Immunological study of cerebral senile amyloid (congophilic angiopathy and senile plaques). Interdisc Top Gerontol 19: 127–130

Stam FC, Rozemuller JM, Eikelenboom P. Immunopathological aspects of senile brain amyloidosis. In: Pepeu G et al. (eds) New trends in aging research. Sirmione, Italy, in press

Tavolato B, Argentiero V, (1980) Immunological indices in presenile Alzheimer's disease. J Neurol Sci 46: 325–331

Torack RM, Lynch RG (1981) Cytochemistry of brain amyloid in adult dementia. Acta Neuropathol (Berl) 53: 189–196

Williams A, Papadopoulos N, Chase TN (1980) Demonstration of CSF gamma-globulin banding in presenile dementia. Neurology 30: 882–884

Wisniewski HM, Kozlowski PB (1982) Evidence of blood brain barrier changes in senile dementia of the Alzheimer type. Ann NY Acad Sci 396: 119–129

Wisniewski HM, Merz GS (1983) Neuritic and amyloid plaques in senile dementia of the Alzheimer type. In: Katzman R (ed) Biological aspects of Alzheimer's disease, Banbury report 15, Cold Spring Harbor, New York, pp 145–152

Wisiniewski HM, Terry RD (1973) Reexamination of the pathogenesis of the senile plaque. In: Zimmermann HM (ed) Progress in neuropathology, vol II. Grune and Stratton, New York, pp 1–6

Wisniewski HM, Moretz RC, Lossinsky AS (1981) Evidence for induction of localized amyloid deposits and neuritic plaques by an infectious agent. Ann Neurol 10: 517–522

Wisniewski HM, Lossinsky AS, Moretz RC, Vorbrodt AW, Lassmann H, Carp RI (1983) Increased blood-brain barrier permeability in scrapie-infected mice. J Neuropathol Exp Neurol 42: 615–626

Ultrastructural Study of Senile Plaques and Microvessels in the Brain in Alzheimer's Disease

T. Miyakawa

Summary

Several kinds of senile plaques were examined by light and electron microscopy.

Amyloid masses around capillaries formed the cores of typical senile plaques. All the senile plaques contained at least some amyloid fibrils, and these seemed to be produced at the basement membranes of capillary endothelial cells and projected into the surrounding parenchyma. Even when the senile plaques themselves appeared with light microscopy to lack amyloid fibrils, at least one degenerable capillary with amyloid fibrils was demonstrated when serial sections were examined ultrastructurally. The capillaries producing amyloid fibrils showed degeneration and some of them were destroyed.

The findings described above suggest that the amyloid fibrils which form the cores of several kinds of senile plaques seem to be produced at the basement membrane of the endothelial cell. It is speculated that the capillary degeneration with formation of amyloid fibrils may be a primary change in the genesis of senile plaques.

On the other hand, endothelial cells of many microvessels showed swelling or atrophy, and the basement membranes were hypertrophic and irregular in shape. Considering the described findings above, it might be suggested that the microcirculatory disturbance due to degeneration of the microvessels, including amyloid angiopathy, is very important in the changes in the brain with Alzheimer's disease.

Finally, amyloid fibrils appeared as a rod which was hollow in the center and was composed of a filament arranged as a tightly coiled helix, each turn of which consisted of five globular subunits. This finding showed a new ultrastructure of amyloid fibrils in the brain.

Introduction

Recently, dementia due to Alzheimer's disease has been attracting keen interest because of the social problems ensuing from the disorder. It has been pointed out that numerous senile plaques and neurofibrillary changes are characteristic findings in the brain of patients with Alzheimer's disease. Several theories have been proposed regarding the mechanism of senile plaque production. Although there have been many reports describing senile plaques, the mechanisms by which they are produced have not yet been clearly identified.

This article reports a detailed morphological examination of several kinds of senile plaques made using serial sections for both light and electron microscopes in order to observe the relationship between senile plaques and microvessels. In addition, senile plaques and microvessels were examined by scanning electron microscopy, and replicas of amyloid fibrils produced by a quick-freezing method were examined by electron microscopy.

Material and Methods

The study was carried out on the brains of eight cases of Alzheimer's disease and one case of Down's syndrome. The clinical and histopathological findings were entirely consistent with the diagnosis given. Parts of the cerebral cortex such as temporal lobe, Ammon's horn, and occipital lobe were removed from the brains of the eight patients immediately after death, cut into small pieces and immersed in 3% glutaraldehyde in phosphate buffer (pH 7.4) for 2 h. They were washed in phosphate buffer (pH 7.4) for 10 min, then immersed for 2 h in 2.5% osmium tetroxide in phosphate buffer (pH 7.4). The tissues were dehydrated in alcohol and embedded in epon. Five blocks were selected from each part of the brain and serial sections were stained with toluidine blue for light microscopy. Then 200 sheet meshes of serial thin sections (30–50 nm) were taken from each block of each case examined. They were stained with uranyl acetate and lead solutions or alkaline bismuth solution, and examined with a Hitachi 12A electron microscope (100 kV). In the serial sections, 90 senile plaques were thoroughly examined, and thick sections (300–500 nm) were also examined with a Jeol 2000 Ex (200 kV) electron microscope.

In addition, in each case, 300 serial sections, 5 µm thick, were cut from the paraffin blocks and stained with silver and PAS solution for examination by light microscopy. Then parts of the cerebral cortex were removed, cut into small pieces, and immersed in 3% glutaraldehyde in phosphate buffer (pH 7.4) for 3 h. They were washed in distilled water for 15 min then frozen in liquefied nitrogen and immediately cracked. These tissues were treated with 8 NHCl for 15 min at 60° C, then washed in distilled water for 20 min. They were immersed in 2.5% osmium tetroxide for 2 h then dehydrated and dried by the critical point method, and, after being coated with platinum, were examined with a Hitachi S310 electron microscope.

The fresh material from the brain affected with Down's syndrome was cut into small pieces and immersed in 2% formaldehyde for 12 h and was used for producing replicas by a quick-freezing method (Heuser et al. 1979). The replicas were also examined with the Jeol 200 EX (200 kV) electron microscope. For examination of the blood vessels in the brain, only those separated and gathered from the brain by means of the ultrasonic method were examined with electron microscopy.

Results

Light Microscopical Findings

When preparations are examined with silver stain, two kinds of senile plaques are seen: a typical senile plaque (Fig. 1a) having a central core of amyloid mass, and a

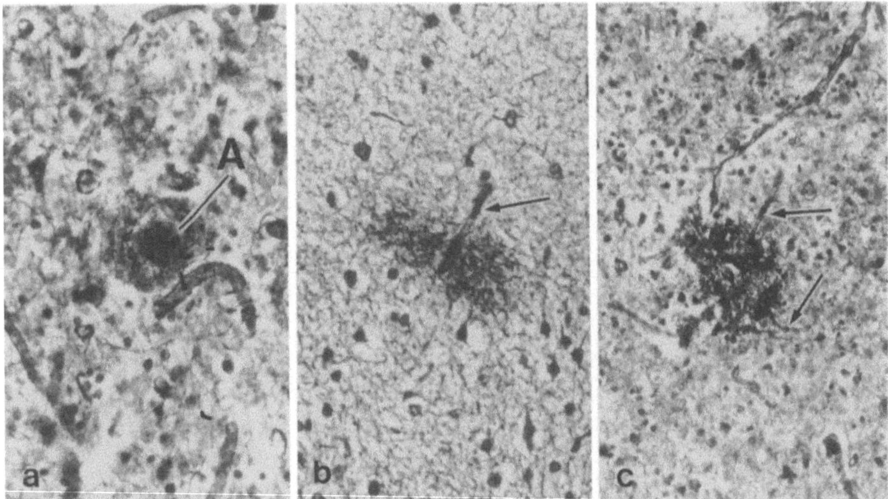

Fig. 1a–c. a Typical senile plaque which has a central core of amyloid mass (*A*). Silver stain, × 700.
b Primitive senile plaque. A capillary (*arrow*) passes through the senile plaque. Silver stain, × 330.
c Primitive senile plaque which is in close relation to capillaries (*arrows*). Silver stain, × 250

primitive senile plaque (Fig. 1b, c) without a central core of amyloid mass. Some of the plaques had a close relationship to microvessels (Fig. 1b, c).

Examining serial sections with PAS stain, almost all of the senile plaques, or amyloid deposits forming the central cores of senile plaques, had a close relationship with the capillaries (Fig. 2). Also, in the serial sections with toluidine blue stain obtained from epon blocks, all of the amyloid masses forming the central cores of typical senile plaques were amyloid deposited around small blood vessels (Fig. 3a–c). However, very few senile plaques could be said to lack any relationship to microvessels.

Loss of nerve cells and degeneration of nerve cells were diffusely observed, independent of senile plaques and Alzheimer's neurofibrillary tangles, in the cortices of the brains.

Electron Microscopical Findings

Examination by light microscopy of typical senile plaques that were in close relation to microvessels showed that amyloid masses consisting of amyloid fibrils always existed around capillaries. The numerous amyloid fibrils projected directly from the capillaries with amyloid angiopathy into the surrounding parenchyma (Fig. 4). In serial sections, amyloid fibrils projected from the capillary basement membrane areas into senile plaques (Fig. 5a), and at other points these same capillaries exhibited changes of amyloid angiopathy. Here, numerous amyloid fibrils projected into the surround-

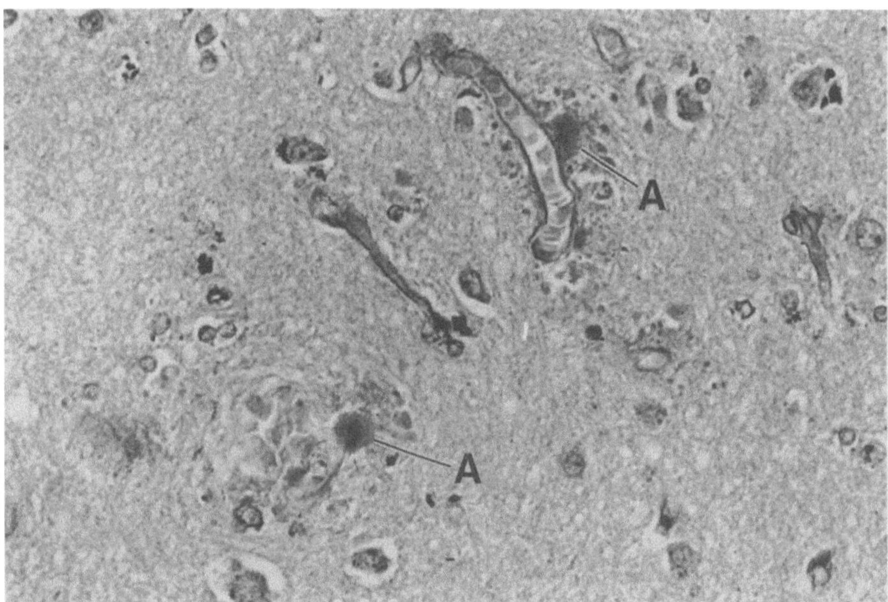

Fig. 2. Amyloid masses (A) around capillaries form the central core of typical senile plaques. PAS stain, × 480

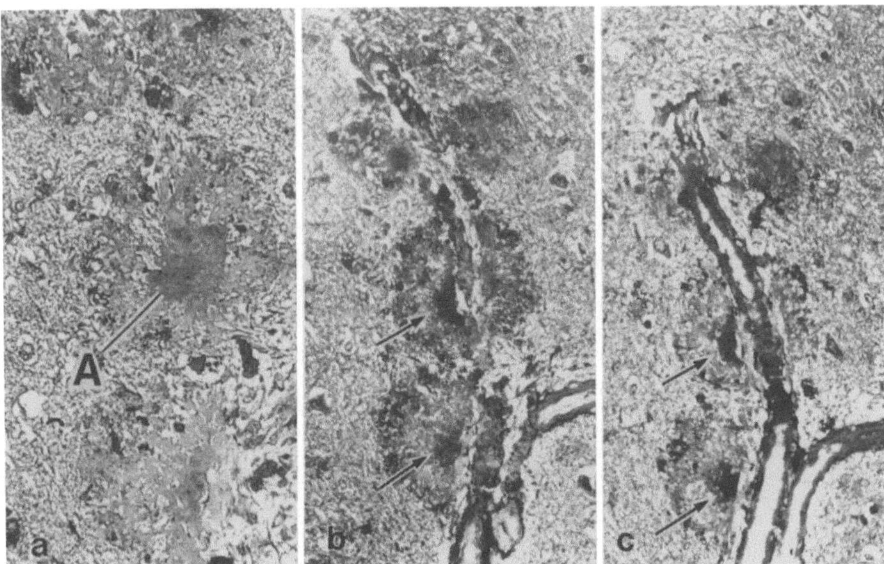

Fig. 3a–c. Serial sections with toluidine blue stain. **a** Typical senile plaque having a core of amyloid mass (A) does not seem to be related to a blood vessel. × 650. **b** Degenerated small blood vessel passes through senile plaques. Amyloid deposits (*arrows*) around the blood vessel exist in the center of the senile plaque. × 365. **c** Senile plaques attach themselves to the back of a small blood vessel. *Arrows*, amyloid mass. × 365

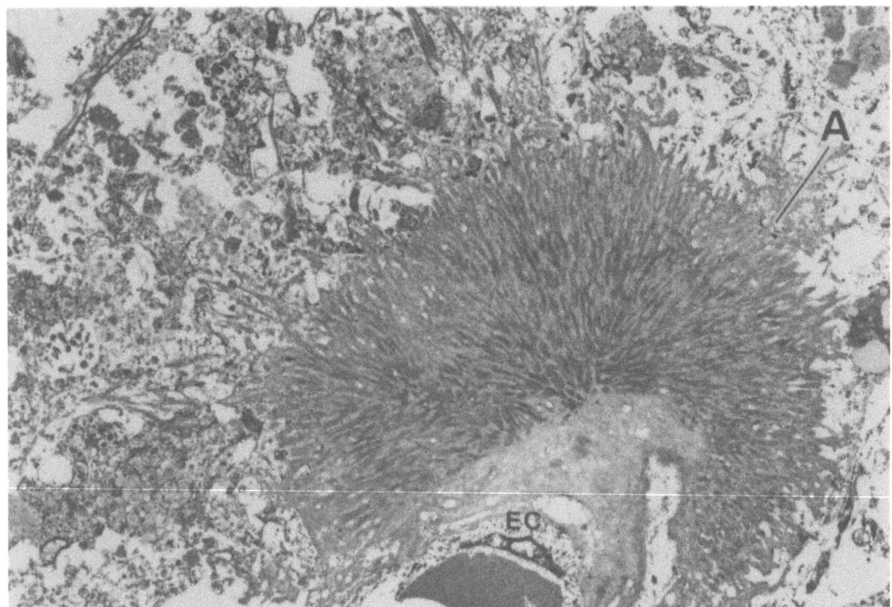

Fig. 4. Amyloid mass (*A*), consisting of amyloid fibrils, directly attaches to a degenerated capillary with amyloid angiopathy. This shows that numerous amyloid fibrils project into the surrounding parenchyma from the capillary. *EC,* endothelial cell, × 2600

ing parenchyma and formed the cores of typical senile plaques. The endothelial cells were swollen and were being destroyed (Fig. 5b).

Even when senile plaques seemed to have no relationship with the capillaries under a light microscope, electron microscopy invariably demonstrated at least one degenerated or destroyed capillary with amyloid angiopathy (Fig. 6). However, it was only by the use of serial sections that the capillaries could be identified as such, since, as they were being destroyed, their lumens became filled with debris formed from destroyed endothelial cells.

In specimens of 300–500 nm thickness, observed using the 200-kV electron microscope, the amyloid masses seen around the capillaries by light microscopy consisted of numerous amyloid fibrils spreading as a radial structure from the wall of the blood vessels to the parenchyma (Fig. 7). Even in primitive senile plaques, amyloid fibrils spread from the capillary walls into the surrounding parenchyma (Fig. 8). Examining the amyloid fibrils projecting from capillaries in thin sections, the fibrils seemed to be produced in the capillary basement membranes (Fig. 9). Where the senile plaques cracked, rough solid substances containing degenerated cell processes were observed, and degenerated capillaries passed through them (Fig. 10).

Examination of replicas of amyloid fibrils made by the quick freezing method showed the fiber to have a hollow structure with a diameter of 13–15 nm. It consisted of a tightly coiled helix, each turn of which appeared to be composed of five globular

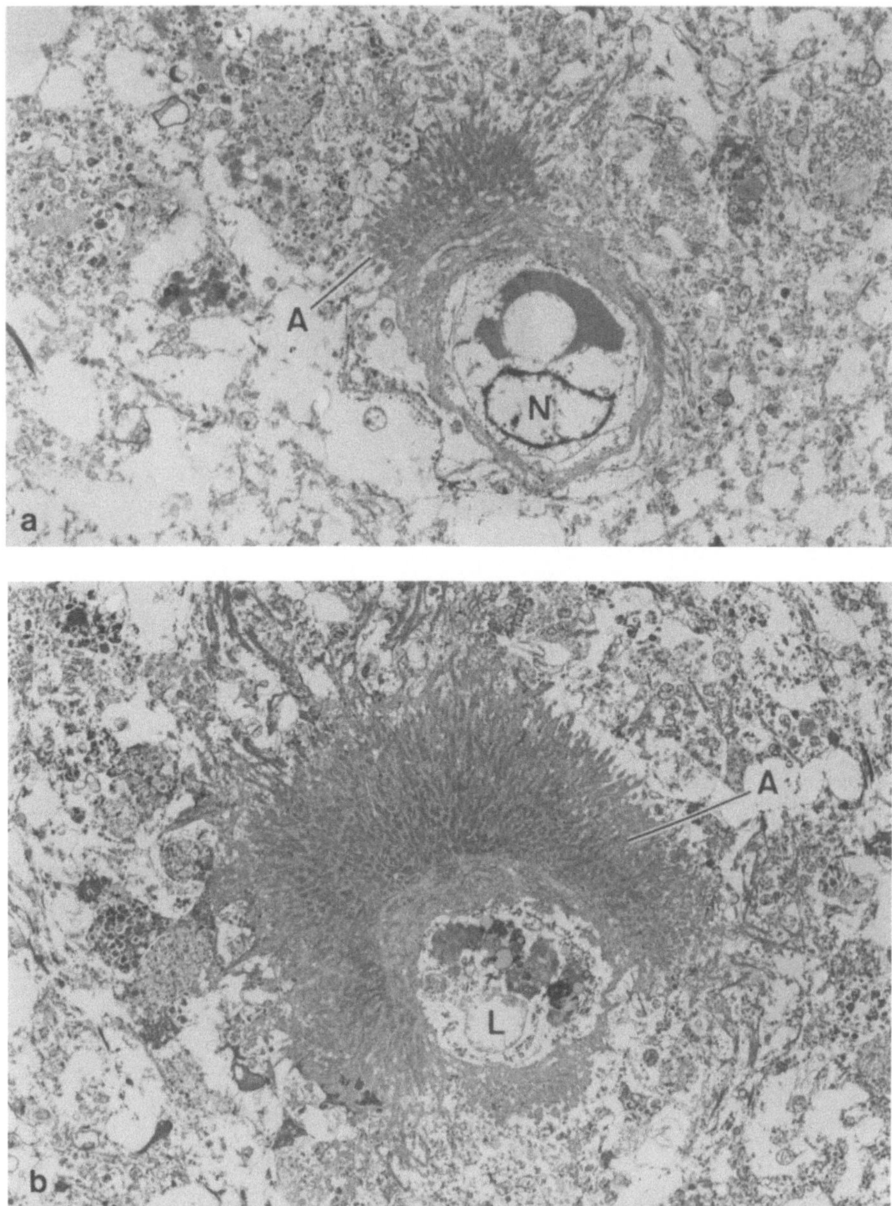

Fig. 5a–b. Serial sections of a typical senile plaque. **a** Amyloid fibrils (*A*) project directly from the wall of a capillary with amyloid angiopathy into parenchyma. *N*, nucleus of endothelial cell, × 3600. **b** Amyloid mass (*A*), forming the central core of a typical senile plaque, surrounds a degenerated endothelial cell which contains many lysosome-like bodies. The lumen (*L*) of the capillary is narrowed. × 4100

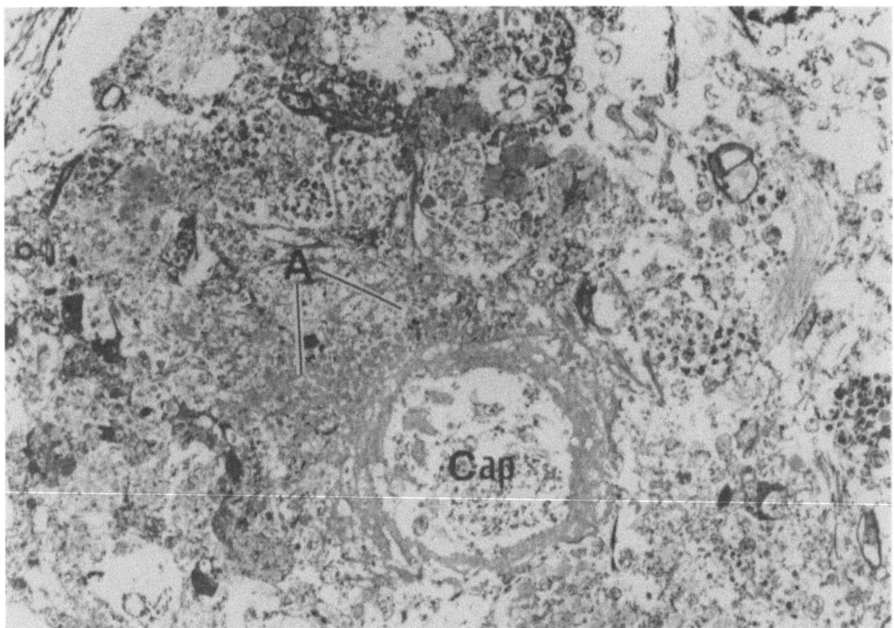

Fig. 6. Primitive senile plaque. The lumen of a capillary (*Cap*) is filled with debris from a destroyed endothelial cell. Many amyloid fibrils (*A*) project from the capillary and extend into senile plaque. × 4100

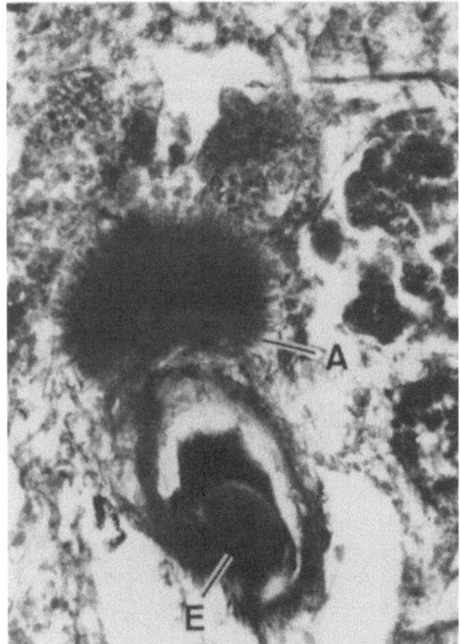

Fig. 7. Central core of amyloid mass (*A*) around a capillary obtained from a thick section. Amyloid fibrils project from the wall of the capillary into parenchyma. *E*, erythrocyte. × 3360

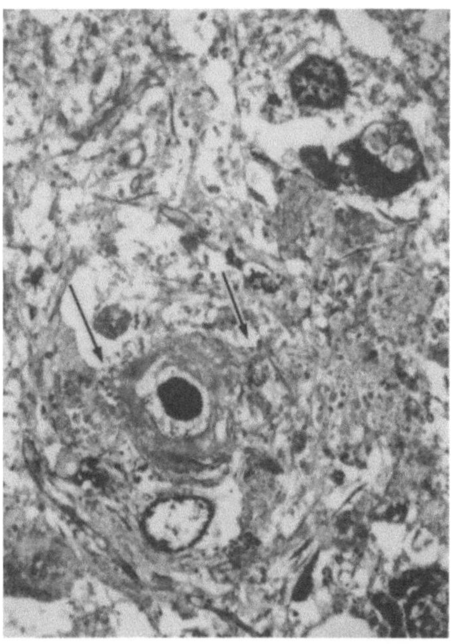

Fig. 8. Primitive senile plaque obtained from a thick section contains a destroyed capillary with amyloid angiopathy. Amyloid fibrils (*arrows*) spread into the primitive senile plaque. × 2000

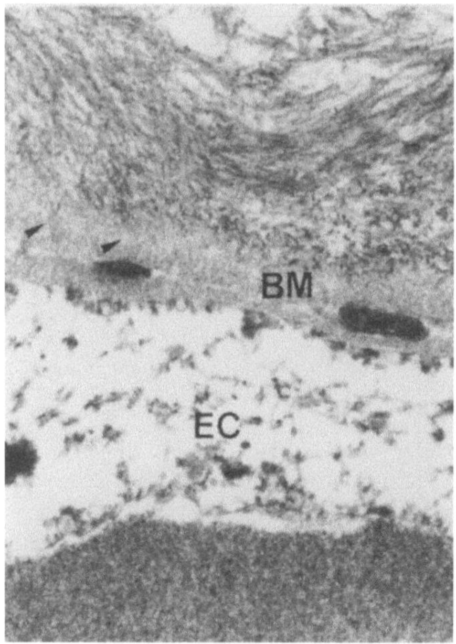

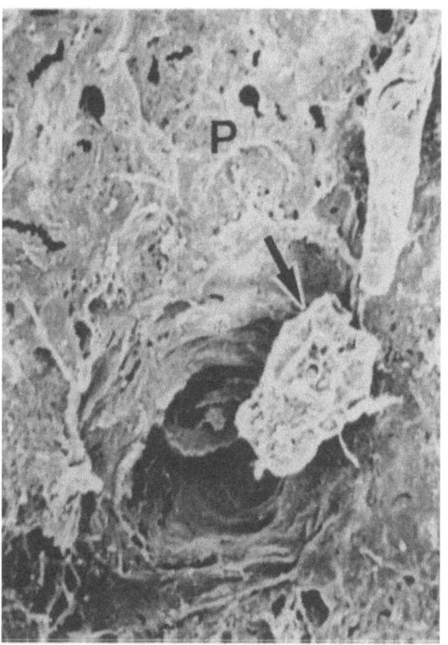

Fig. 9. Part of a capillary. Amyloid fibrils (*arrowheads*) apparently appear in the basement membrane (*BM*). *EC*, endothelial cell. × 65000

Fig. 10. Cracked surface through a senile plaque obtained with a scanning electron microscope. Rough solid substances which contained degenerated cell processes surround degenerated capillary (*arrow*). *P*, senile plaque. × 1900

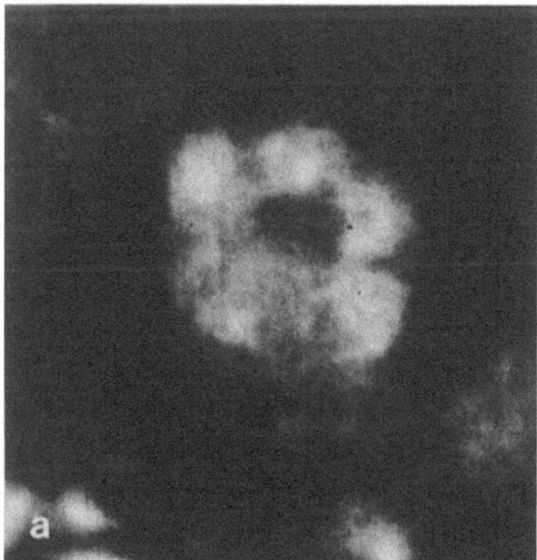

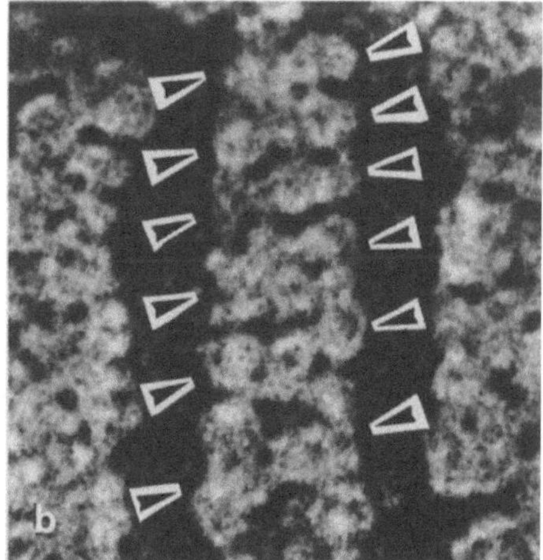

Fig. 11a, b. **a** Replica of amyloid fibril in a transverse direction. One turn of helix consists of about five globular subunits. × 1600000. **b** Replica of amyloid fibril in a longitudinal direction. Each subunit (3–5 nm) is arrayed in a helical form (*arrowheads*). × 1344000

subunits, each having a width of 3–5 nm (Fig. 11a). The subunits were attached to each other and arranged in a helix (Fig. 11b).

From the above findings, a structural model of an amyloid fibril can be made (Fig. 12).

In the areas without senile plaque, many microvessels showed degeneration of endothelial cells and pericytes. The basement membranes of the capillaries were hypertrophic and irregular in shape (Fig. 13). In some capillaries, the lumen was occluded (Fig. 14).

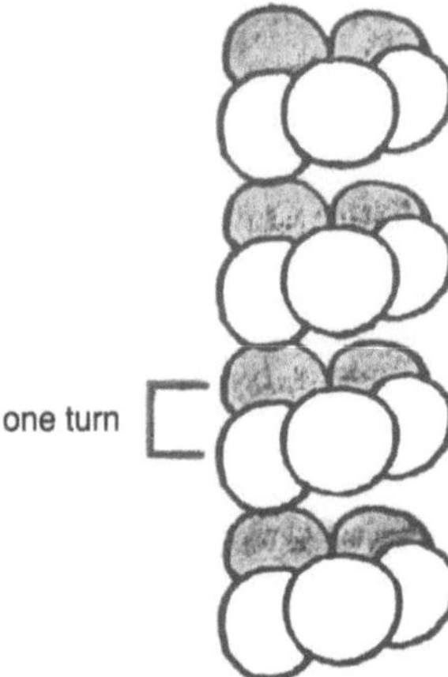

Fig. 12. Structural model of an amyloid fibril

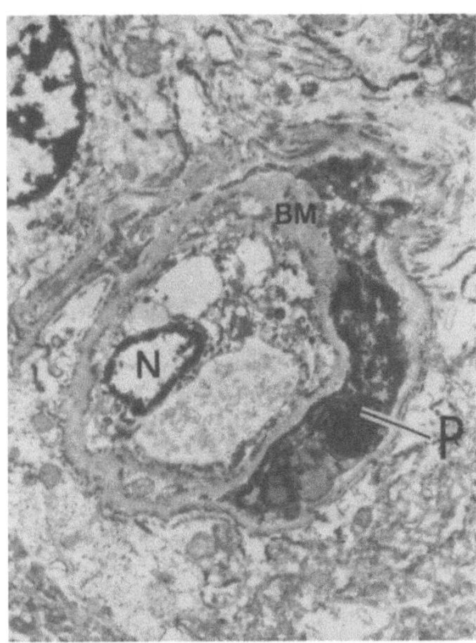

Fig. 13. Capillary. The basement membrane (*MB*) is thickened and tortuous. Endothelial cell and pericyte (*P*) show degeneration. *N*, nucleus of endothelial cell. × 5200

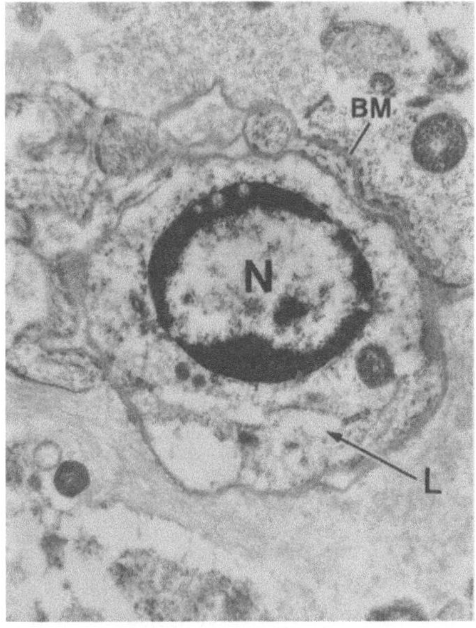

Fig. 14. Capillary. The basement membrane (*BM*) is thickened and tortuous. The endothelial cell is hypertrophic and the lumen (*L*) is narrowed and obstructed. *N*, nucleus of endothelial cell. × 16000

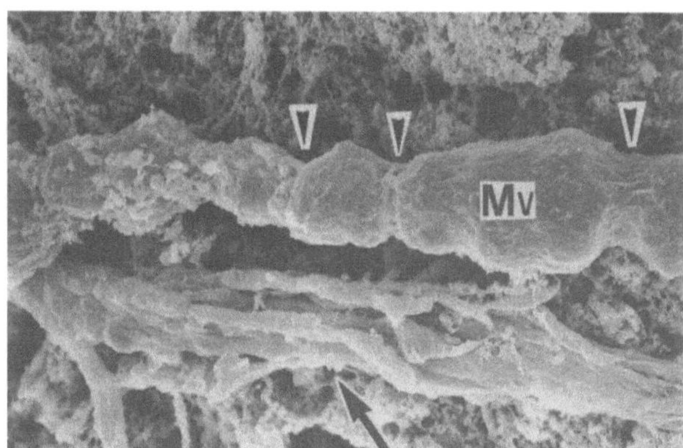

Fig. 15. Microvessel (*Mv*) and capillaries (*arrow*). Precapillary arteriole microvessel shows a series of focal constrictions (*arrowheads*) and many capillaries are arranged in a bundle. × 1600

The examination of the blood vessels obtained by the ultrasonic method showed the microvessels to have a series of focal constrictions, and many capillaries were arranged in a bundle (Fig. 15).

Discussion

Since Alzheimer (1907) first observed abundant senile plaques in the brains of patients with Alzheimer's disease and senile dementia, senile plaques have been considered characteristic of Alzheimer's disease. Many morphological studies on the mechanism of senile plaque production have been reported to date; however, the exact mechanisms by which they are formed have not yet been clearly identified.

Scholz (1938) reported plaque-like degeneration of arteries and capillaries („drusige Entartung der Hirnarterien") and concluded that the core of senile plaques consisted of material which permeated from the blood vessels. Morel and Wildi (1952) reported that the aged had paraproteinemia which influenced the capillaries to produce senile plaque. Other authors have described similar findings (Corsellis and Brierly 1954; Pantelakis 1954; Yokoi and Ishii 1958; Ishii 1969).

In 1961, Surbeck reported "dyshoric angiopathy" following senile plaques. Mandybur (1967) reported that there was a correlation between the presence of amyloid-rich plaques and cerebral amyloid angiopathy (especially the plaque-like angiopathy) but that this had no correlation with "amyloid-poor" senile plaques.

Schlote (1965) reported that plaque-like angiopathy results from the infiltration of vessels by certain plasma proteins and electron micrographs of affected vessels show amyloid fibrils arranged in "brush-like structures" on the adventitial surface. This may indicate a transmural flow of "precursor" substances through the vessels to the cerebral parenchyma. Glenner (1979) reported that, in a large proportion of cases of Alzheimer's presenile dementia, the major causal mechanism was an alteration of the blood-brain barrier resulting from the deposition of Congo red-positive material in the walls of small blood vessels occurring at a relatively young age. He concluded that a partially digested, filamentous protein (filarin) is further cleaved enzymatically by microglial cells to produce the amyloid core of the neurite plaque.

On the other hand, Friede and Magee (1962) found 92% of senile plaques (probably neuritic) to be unrelated to capillaries. Thus, amyloids may be found in various locations in the brain without degenerating neurites, although large clusters of these neurites are always accompanied by amyloids. Wisniewski and Terry (1973) concluded that the origin of the classic plaque lies in the degeneration of neurites which precedes the deposition of amyloid. Recently, Wisniewski et al. (1981) considered the pathogenesis of amyloid fibril and senile plaque production. They reported that amyloid deposits in all areas were closely associated with rod-shaped or oval cells, rich in free and membrane-bound ribosomes, and containing a distended endoplasmic reticulum. With both light and electron microscopy, these amyloid-associated cells appeared to be reactive microglial cells.

By contrast, we noted the presence of amyloid fibrils around the blood vessels with amyloid angiopathy in the senile plaques (Miyakawa et al. 1974; Miyakawa and Uehara 1979; Miyakawa et al. 1982; Miyakawa 1986) and were certain that all the senile plaques contained at least some amyloid fibrils, which seemed to be produced at the basement membranes of capillary endothelial cells and spread into surrounding parenchyma. Even when senile plaques themselves appeared to lack amyloid fibrils when examined using light microscopy, at least one degenerable capillary containing amyloid fibrils was demonstrable when serial sections were examined ultrastructurally. We suggested that all the amyloids forming the core of senile plaques have an intimate relationship with the capillary and that several kinds of senile plaques seem to be the result of a primary change in the capillary involving the formation of amyloid fibrils.

We found many degenerated neurites without so-called amyloid-producing cells. As is well known, amyloid masses forming the core of senile plaques consist of numerous amyloid fibrils. If the masses are produced by amyloid-producing cells, many of these cells should be observable; however, from our observations, they could hardly be seen, even by electron microscopy.

Following the findings described above, we examined thick sections by electron microscopy. The results obtained confirmed those obtained from thin sections. The findings described above might help elucidate the mechanism of the morphological production of amyloid fibrils and senile plaques.

Recently, Glenner and Wong (1984a, b) found a unique cerebrovascular amyloid fibril protein in the serum in patients with Alzheimer's disease and with Down's syndrome. This finding is highly relevant to cerebrovascular changes with amyloid angiopathy and is closely linked to our morphological findings.

The ultrastructure of amyloid fibrils in the brain has not yet been examined. Shirahama and Cohen (1967) examined amyloid-laden tissues (spleen and liver) and reported that the amyloid filaments are approximately 7.5–8 nm in diameter and consist of five subunits. Glenner et al. (1968) also examined the human spleen, liver and kidney containing amyloid deposits and detected the two morphological components of human amyloid deposits, the periodic rod and fibril. The periodic rods were up to 250 nm in length, and small unit structures were approximately 9 nm in diameter. The fibrils were aggregations of 7,5–8 nm filaments devoid of a periodic rod. According to our findings, using the replicas of amyloid fibrils produced by the quick-freezing method, the amyloid fibril showed a rod which was hollow in the center and was composed of a filament arranged as a tightly coiled helix, each turn of which consisted of five globular subunits (Miyakawa et al. 1986a, b). This showed a new ultrastructure of amyloid fibril in the brain.

Nonspecific changes such as atrophy and loss of the nerve cells observed diffusely in the cortex must be considered the most important findings in the brains of patients with Alzheimer's disease. These changes might be directly related to clinical symptoms, especially dementia. Not much interest has been shown in these nonspecific changes although, as was shown by this study, small blood vessels and capillaries in parts of slightly damaged cortices showed signs of degeneration. A great number of endothelial cells of microvessels were swollen or atrophic, and the basement membranes of the microvessels were hypertrophic and irregular in shape. The pericytes had also degenerated and glial feet surrounding these microvessels were swollen. Scanning electron microscopy revealed that the microvessels had an abnormal shape.

Taking these findings into consideration, it seemed the initial changes in the histopathological findings were a microcirculatory disturbance of the brain due to change or degeneration of the microvessels. The changes in the microvessels were, over a long period, likely to induce the disturbance in the exchange of the blood substances between the blood vessels and the parenchyma. These nonspecific changes in the nerve cells diffusely observed in the cortices of the brain might be secondarily induced by the change in the blood vessels. Severe dementia observed in Alzheimer's disease and senile dementia were consistent with the pathological changes in a great number of the nerve cells with nonspecific changes. From this it might be strongly suggested that the microcirculatory disturbance due to degeneration of the microvessels, including amyloid angiopathy, plays an important role in the primary change in the brain affected by Alzheimer's disease.

Lassen et al. (1960) and Ingvar et al. (1968) described the reductions of cerebral blood flow and cerebral oxygen consumption in presenile and senile dementia.

In addition, the disturbance of the blood-brain barrier induced by amyloid angiopathy seems to play an important role in the pathological mechanism of Alzheimer's disease (Nandy 1978; Glenner et al. 1981; Friedland et al. 1983). Matsushita (1986) reported that the regions most severely damaged in the brain with Alzheimer's disease are parts of the watershed areas in the arteries, and that the extent of pathological changes might be influenced by blood flow. The findings described above suggest degeneration of the microvessels, including amyloid angiopathy, may play a crucial part in the pathogenesis of Alzheimer's disease.

Finally, I would like to strongly emphasize that disturbances of microvessels provide a vital clue as to the pathogenesis of Alzheimer's disease.

References

Alzheimer A (1907) Über eigenartige Erkrankung der Hirnrinde. Allg Z Psychiatr 64: 146–148
Corsellis JAN, Brierly JB (1954) An unusual type of presenile dementia. Brain 77: 571–587
Friede RL, Magee KR (1962) Alzheimer's disease: presentation of a case with pathologic and enzymatic-histochemical observations. Neurology 12: 213–222
Friedland RP, Yano Y, Budinger TF, Ganz E, Husesmann RH, Derenzo SE, Knittle B (1983) Quantitative evaluation of blood brain barrier integrity in Alzheimer's type dementia. Positron emission tomographic studies with rubidium 82. Neurology 22 (Suppl 2): 19
Glenner GG (1979) Congophilic microangiopathy in the pathogenesis of Alzheimer's syndrome (presenile dementia). Med Hypotheses 5: 1231–1236

Glenner GG, Wong CW (1984a) Alzheimer's disease: Initial purification and characterization of a novel cerebrovascular amyloid protein. Biochem Biophys Res Commun 122: 885–890

Glenner GG, Wong CW (1984b) Alzheimer's disease and Down's syndrome: Sharing of a unique cerebrovascular amyloid fibril protein. Biochem Biophys Res Commun 122: 1131–1135

Glenner GG, Keiser HR, Bladen HA, Cuatrecasas P, Eanes ED, Ram JS, Kanfer JN, Delellis RA (1968) Amyloid. VI. A comparison of two morphologic components of human amyloid deposits. J Histochem Cytochem 16: 633–644

Glenner GG, Henry JH, Fujihara S (1981) Congophilic angiopathy in the pathogenesis of Alzheimer's degeneration. Ann Pathol 1: 120–129

Heuser JE, Reese TS, Dennis MJ, Jan Y, Jan L (1979) Synaptic vesicle exocytosis captured by quick freezing and correlated with quantal transmitter release. J Cell Biol 81: 275–300

Ingvar DH, Obist W, Chirian E, Cronquist S, Risberg J, Gustafson L, Hagerdal M, Wittbom-Cigern G (1968) General and regional abnormalities of cerebral blood flow in senile and presenile dementia. Scand J Clin Lab Invest [Suppl] 102: X11 B

Ishii T (1969) Enzyme histochemical studies of senile plaques and the plaque-like degeneration of arteries and capillaries (Scholz). Acta Neuropathol 14: 250–260

Lassen NA, Feinberg I, Lane MH (1960) Bilateral studies of cerebral oxygen uptake in young and aged normal subjects and in patients with organic dementia. J Clin Invest 29: 491–500

Mandybur TI (1967) The incidence of cerebral amyloid angiopathy in Alzheimer's disease. Neurology 25: 120–125

Matsushita M (1986) Morphological speciality in Alzheimer's disease. Clin Neurol (Jpn) 26: 1283–1285

Miyakawa T (1986) The relationship between amyloid fibrils around cerebral blood vessels and senile plaques, and ultrastructure of amyloid fibrils. International symposium on dementia and amyloid (Tokyo, Japan). Neuropathology (Suppl 3): 37–48

Miyakawa T, Uehara Y (1979) Observations of amyloid angiopathy and senile plaques by the scanning electron miroscope. Acta Neuropathol (Berl) 48: 153–156

Miyakawa T, Sumiyoshi S, Murayama E, Deshimaru M (1974) Ultrastructure of capillary plaque-like degeneration in senile dementia. Mechanism of amyloid production. Acta Neuropathol (Berl) 29: 229–236

Miyakawa T, Shimoji A, Kuramoto R, Higuchi Y (1982) The relationship between senile plaques and cerebral blood vessels in Alzheimer's disease and senile dementia. Morphological mechanism of senile plaque production. Virchows Arch [B] 40: 121–129

Miyakawa T, Katsuragi S, Watanabe K, Shimoji A, Ikeuchi Y (1986a) Ultrastructural studies of amyloid fibrils and senile plaques in human brain. Acta Neuropathol 70: 202–208

Miyakawa T, Watanabe K, Katsuragi S (1986b) Ultrastructure of amyloid fibrils in Alzheimer's disease and Down's syndrome. Virchows Arch [B] 52: 99–106

Morel F, Wildi E (1952) General and cellular pathochemistry of senile and presenile alterations of the brain. Proceedings of the 1st international congress of neuropathology, Rome. Casa Editrice Libreria, Rosenberg and Sellier, Turin, pp 347–374

Nandy K (1978) Alzheimer's disease. In: Katzman R et al. (eds) Aging (workshop conference), No 7. Raven, New York, p 505

Pantelakis S (1954) Un type particulier d'angiopathie senile du systeme nerveaux central: l'angiopathie congophilie. Topographie et frequences. Monatsschr Psychiatr Neurol 198: 219–256

Schlote W (1965) Die Amyloidnatur der kongophilen, drusigen Entartung der Hirnarterien (Scholz) im Senium. Acta Neuropathol (Berl) 4: 449–468

Scholz W (1938) Studien zur Pathologie der Hirngefäße in Senium. Proceedings of the 5th international congress of neuropathology, Zurich. pp 490–494

Shirahama T, Cohen AS (1967) High-resolution electron microscopic analysis of the amyloid fibrils. J Cell Biol 33: 679–708

Surbeck KB (1961) L'angiopathie dyshorique (Morel) de l'ecorce cerebrale. Etude anatomoclinique et statistique. Aspect genetique. Thesis, University of Geneva

Wisniewski H, Terry RD (1973) Reexamination of the pathogenesis of the senile plaque. Prog Neuropathol 11: 1–26

Wisniewski H, Moretz R, Lossinsky A (1981) Evidence for induction of localized amyloid deposits and neurite plaques by an infectious agent. Ann Neurol 10: 517–522

Yokoi S, Ishii T (1958) Histochemistry of plaque-like degeneration in the brain of senile dementia. Psychiatr Neurol (Jpn) 60: 641–649

Paired Helical Filaments in Alzheimer's Disease: Their Formation and Transformation

A. Delacourte, and *A. Defossez*

Summary

The formation and degradation mechanisms of paired helical filaments (PHF) are still unclear. A study of these phenomena was undertaken using a specific anti-PHF immune serum.

Tau proteins are the major antigenic components of PHF (as demonstrated by immunoblotting and immunocytochemistry using anti-PHF and anti-tau immune-sera). Moreover, we have studied the distribution of tau proteins in the different regions of a normal human brain. The anti-PHF strongly detected tau proteins on immunoblots of protein extracts from cortical gray matter, but these proteins were weakly labeled in cortical white matter extracts and almost absent in spinal cord extracts. This distribution of tau proteins, essentially in cortical gray matter of human normal brain, correlates well with the distribution of PHF-containing structures (neurofibrillary tangles, NFT) and degenerating neurites at the periphery of senile plaques (SP) in the cortex with Alzheimer's disease.

Using simultaneous immunolabeling of PHF and elective staining of amyloid deposits by thioflavine, the relationships between PHF and the amyloid substance were studied. Degenerating neurites containing PHF are concentrated like a sleeve around certain pathological vessels with amyloid angiopathy (PHF/AA lesions). PHF/AA lesions seem to be formed by a toxic material brought from blood vessels, leading to the degeneration of surrounding neurites in their close vicinity and provoking the aggregation of tau proteins in PHF. The pathogenesis of such lesions is perhaps similar to the formation of SP containing a capillary in their center.

A comparison of the distribution of PHF and amyloid substance was also performed. In neuronal perikaryons, different populations of NFT were observed, strongly immunolabeled and weakly thioflavine-stained tangles or weakly immunolabeled but strongly thioflavine-stained tangles. Ghost tangles, which correspond to disintegrated NFT, were often exclusively thioflavine-stained. Thus, it is likely that NFT progressively acquire the tinctorial amyloid properties. These observations argue for a catabolism of PHF bundles into an amyloid substance which seems different from other amyloid deposits found in the central core of neuritic plaques and vessel walls.

Introduction

The histopathological lesions of Alzheimer's disease are characterized by the accumulation of two ultrastructural elements in the brain, especially in the association cortex and hippocampus, named paired helical filaments (PHF) and amyloid filaments (AF). PHF are intracellular, 10 nm, helical filaments (Kidd 1963) that constitute bundles observed in the perikaryons of degenerating neurons, called neurofibrillary tangles (NFT). They are found in individual neurites widely distributed in the cortical neuropil, and also in degenerating neurites at the periphery of senile (neuritic) plaques (SP). Amyloid filaments are unpaired filaments, 5–9 nm in diameter (Wisniewski and Merz 1983; Miyakawa et al. 1986), which are found essentially in the core of SP and in the vessel walls with congophilic angiopathy. SP, the most characteristic lesions of Alzheimer's disease, are thus heterogeneous extracellular lesions constituted, at a certain stage of their formation or degradation, by PHF and AF. AF are preesent mainly in the center of SP whereas degenerating neurites located at he periphery contain bundles of PHF.

The nature, formation, and significance of PHF and AF are still a matter of debate and raise questions such as:
- is PHF the hallmark of Alzheimer's disease (Foncin and El Hachimi 1986) or is AF (Selkoe et al. 1987) its characteristic?
- Has the nature of PHF been completely determined (Selkoe 1986)?
- Is the origin of the amyloid substance vascular (Glenner 1983) or neuronal (Masters et al. 1985)?

We have raised a specific anti-PHF immune serum (Persuy et al. 1985) which is an excellent tool for approaching these different problems, especially the study of the formation and transformation of PHF.

The Nature and the Origin of PHF

The composition of PHF

Knowledge about the chemical structure of PHF should shed light on the mechanisms of PHF formation and their pathological significance. Since PHF insolubility makes biochemical analysis extremely difficult, the more rational way to determine the nature of PHF constituents is to raise and characterize specific antibodies against these structures.

Fig. 1a–c. a, b Light micrographs of two adjacent paraffin sections of Alzheimer-affected hippocampus. NFT (*arrows*) and SP (*arrowheads*) are simultaneously immunolabeled by *a* anti-PHF and **b** anti-tau. Bar, 50 μm. **c** Electron micrograph of an ultrathin section of Alzheimer-affected temporal cortex showing double immunogold labeling of PHF by anti-PHF (gold particles 5 nm in diameter, *arrows*) and by anti-tau (gold particles 20 nm in diameter, *arrowheads*). Bar, 0.4 μm. Indirect peroxidase method was performed on paraffin sections as described by Delacourte and Défossez (1986a). Double immunogold labeling was obtained on ultrathin Araldite sections with the postembedding method used by Beauvillain et al. (1984)

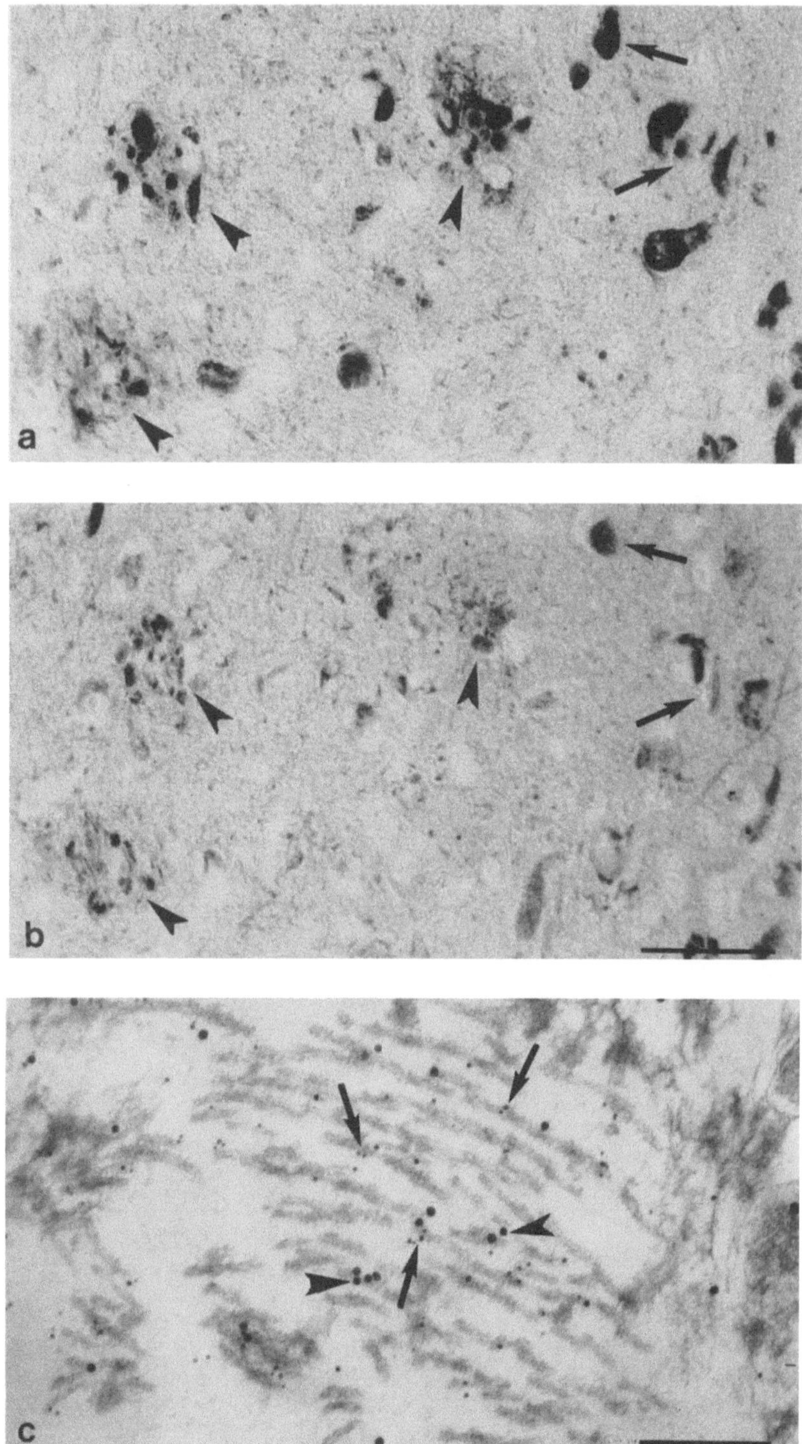

Fig. 1

At the optical level, our anti-PHF immune serum specifically labels NFT and the degenerating neurites surrounding SP on Alzheimer-affected cortex sections. Approximately 50 brains and ten biopsies have been analyzed and specific immunolabeling of NFT and SP was always obtained, regardless of the fixation technique (formol, Carnoy, Zamboni) or inclusion technique (parafin, cryostat sections, Araldite embedding) used. At the ultrastructural level, PHF are immunolabeled with the antiserum whereas the other cytoplasmic structures are not immunostained (Delacourte and Défossez 1986a,b; Défossez et al. 1987) (Fig. 1).

On immunoblots performed with normal and Alzheimer-affected SDS brain extracts, the anti-PHF exclusively recognized a set of proteins with a molecular weight of 65–45 kd (Fig. 2). This set of proteins corresponds to tau proteins, the promoting factors of microtubule polymerization (Delacourte and Défossez 1986a,b). Moreover, we have raised immunsera against tau proteins (extracted from rat, ox, and human brains) that label NFT and SP at the optical level and PHF at the ultrastructural level (Fig. 1). These results confirm the pioneering work of Brion et al. (1985). Thus, immunoblotting and immunocytochemistry demonstrate that tau proteins are the major components of PHF. Other laboratories published identical conclusions simultaneously (Ihara et al. 1986; Grundke-Iqbal et al. 1986a,b; Kosik et al. 1986; Nukina and Ihara 1986; Wood et al. 1986).

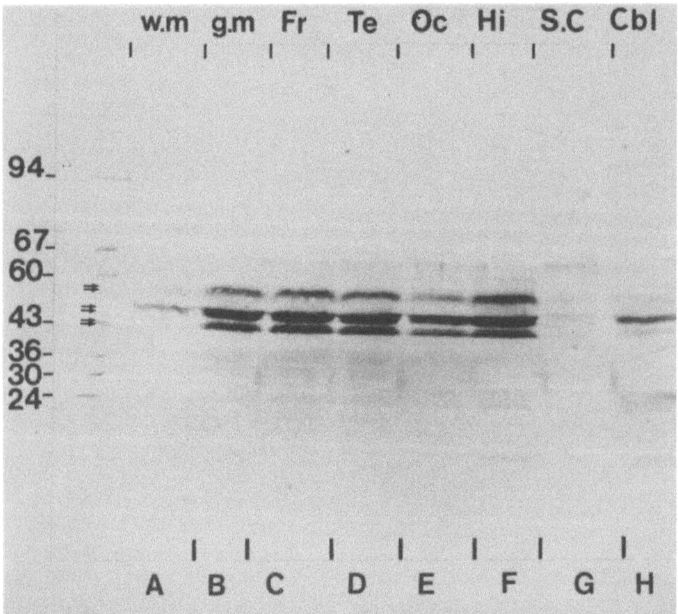

Fig. 2. Quantitative analysis of tau proteins immunodetected by an anti-PHF in the different regions of a normal human brain. Note the strong immunodetection of tau proteins (*arrows*) in the cortical gray matter and its absence in the spinal cord. Each sample of nerve tissue was homogenized in 10 volumes of SDS buffer and 25 µl was loaded. Proteins were resolved by SDS-polyacrylamide gel electrophoresis, transferred on to a nitrocellulose sheet and reacted with the anti-PHF (dilution 1/200) and an antirabbit globulin conjugated with peroxidase. 2-Chloronaphthol staining. *A*, white matter (*w.m*) dissected from temporal cortex; *B*, gray matter (*g.m*) dissected from temporal cortex; *C*, frontal cortex (*Fr*); *D*, temporal cortex (*Te*); *E*, occipital cortex (*Oc*); *F*, hippocampal cortex (*Hi*); *G*, spinal cord (*S.C*); *H*, cerebellum (*Cbl*)

However, the presence of other cytoskeletal components in PHF, especially neurofilament proteins and microtubule-associated protein (MAP2) (Gambetti et al. 1986; Miller et al. 1986; Yen et al. 1987), has also been demonstrated. But, as far as neurofilaments are concerned, these results were obtained with antineurofilament monoclonal antibodies that cross-react with tau and MAP2 phosphorylation sites (Nukina et al. 1987; Ksiezak-Reding et al. 1987). The presence of MAP2 epitopes in the PHF structure may also be due to the known cross-reaction between tau proteins and MAP2 that bind to the same C-terminal part of β-tubulin (Littauer et al. 1986).

In conclusion, all these results suggest that tau proteins are the major components of PHF, or the major antigenic components, since there is also a possibility that nonantigenic components can also be integrated into the PHF structure (Selkoe 1986). The nonantigenic protein to be thus integrated would be the amyloid protein A4 (Masters et al. 1985; Guiroy et al. 1987).

Study of the Distribution of Tau Proteins Detected by the Anti-PHF Immune Serum

Many cytoskeletal proteins have a polarized distribution in the nerve cell related to their function. For example, MAP2 is essentially distributed in dendrites, whereas the P200 neurofilament protein is mainly present in axonal profiles. Therefore, knowledge of the distribution of tau proteins integrated into the PHF structure may provide an insight into their biological role in the normal neuron and also into the mechanisms responsible for the PHF formation.

Using our anti-PHF and anti-tau antisera, we have determined the distribution of these proteins. On immunoblots of resolved SDS protein extracts from different regions of a normal human brain (41 years old), the anti-PHF only detected traces of tau proteins in the dissected cortical white matter, almost none in the spinal cord, and small amounts in the cerebellum. By contrast, large amounts of tau protein were detected in different cortical regions, especially in the dissected cortical gray matter. The different cortical regions studied, i.e., frontal, temporal, occipital, and hippocampus, presented the same immunodetection pattern: five tau proteins of 65–45 kd were immunolabeled (Fig. 2). The immunodetection profile was identical on normal aged brains and was insensitive to the action of alkaline phosphatase.

Thus, tau proteins which were detected with our anti-PHF in the normal brain tissue were distributed essentially in the cortical gray matter. The same results were obtained with polyclonal and monoclonal antibodies against native tau proteins of rat and human origin. The distribution of tau proteins has been studied by other authors with a monoclonal antibody (tau-1) that detects tau proteins in the axons (Binder et al. 1985) and stains Alzheimer lesions (NFT and SP) after their dephosphorylation with alkaline phosphatase (Grundke-Iqbal et al. 1986a). However, in the normal tissue, tau-1 stains axonal structures which are concentrated in the white matter, whereas the Alzheimer lesions are essentially distributed in the gray matter of the associative cortex (layers III and V for NFT; layers II and III for SP).

Therefore, the cortical distribution of tau proteins observed with our anti-PHF correlates well with the distribution of PHF-containing structures (NFT and degenerating neurites at the periphery of SP). This distribution is different from the results obtained with tau-1 which labels a phosphorylation site and probably does not reflect the general distribution of native tau proteins. In conclusion, our results demonstrate that the formation of PHF results from the aggregation of tau proteins normally abundant in the cortical gray matter where the lesions are found in Alzheimer-affected cortex.

The Distribution of PHF Versus AF

Up to now, at the microscopic level, it has been difficult to distinguish between the distribution of PHF and AF, which are sometimes closely intermingled in Alzheimer lesions and often have the same tinctorial affinities due to their β-pleated sheet structure. Silver impregnation stains PHF selectively not staining the amyloid substance of SP and congophilic angiopathy, but it also stains normal neuronal profiles. Nowadays, simultaneous labeling with an anti-PHF and with thioflavine-S (a sensitive marker of amyloid substances) allows a precise comparison of the distribution of immunolabeled PHF with thioflavine-stained amyloid deposits. Using these techniques, we have obtained new information on the composition of Alzheimer lesions that may contribute to the understanding of the formation and degradation of PHF.

The Formation of PHF: Degenerating Neurites Containing PHF are Sometimes Present Around Pathological Blood Vessels

A remarkable morphological relationship between angiopathic blood vessels and degenerating neurites was observed with the simultaneous double-labeling of three brains out of 30 Alzheimer cortices studied. A well-marked concentration of degenerating neurites detected around certain pathological vessels with congophilic angiopathy was visualized with our anti-PHF (Fig. 3). The degenerating neurites were distributed like a sleeve around certain vessels with amyloid angiopathy (AA) (Delacourte et al. 1987) and were named PHF/AA lesions. The degenerating neurites, which were also labeled with anti-tau immune sera and by silver impregnation, are closely intermingled with thioflavine-stained neurites. On serial sections, we followed several vessels with PHF/AA over a length of 1–2 mm. PHF/AA were essentially localized around vessels with a diameter of 60 μm but larger vessels (up to 120 μm) were also observed. On the whole, one in ten of the angiopathic vessels observed on histological sections from different areas of associative cortex showed these PHF/AA lesions.

Since these lesions are rare, it is difficult to make a detailed analysis of their distribution and more information is needed to understand the mechanisms of their formation. However, it is tempting to speculate that these PHF/AA lesions result from a poisoning of neurite endings which pick up toxic material from the disrupted

---

Fig. 3a–c. Double staining of one paraffin section by thioflavine and anti-PHF (bar, 30 μm). Three light micrographs of one vessel with **a** fluorescence optics, **b** bright field optics, and **c** simultaneously with fluorescence optics and low-intensity bright-field optics. Note that the fluorescent vessel wall is not immunolabeled and is surrounded by degenerating neurites, thioflavine stained and/or immunostained

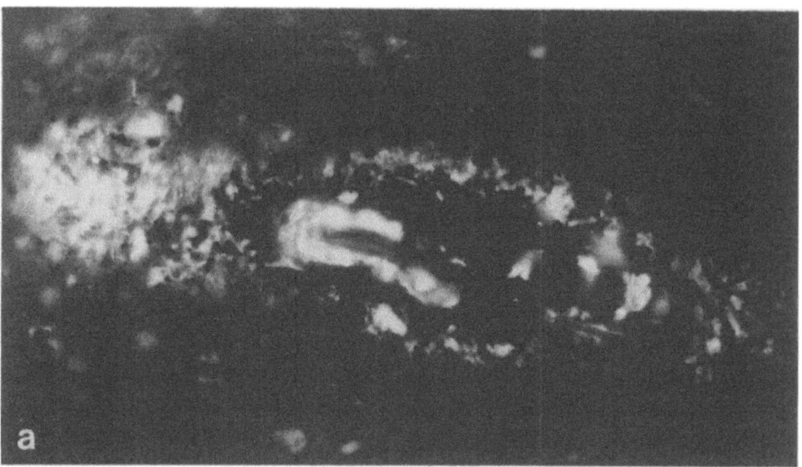

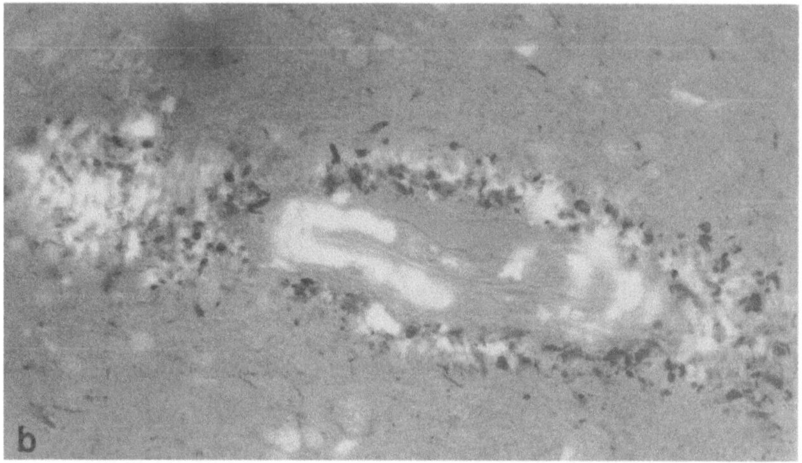

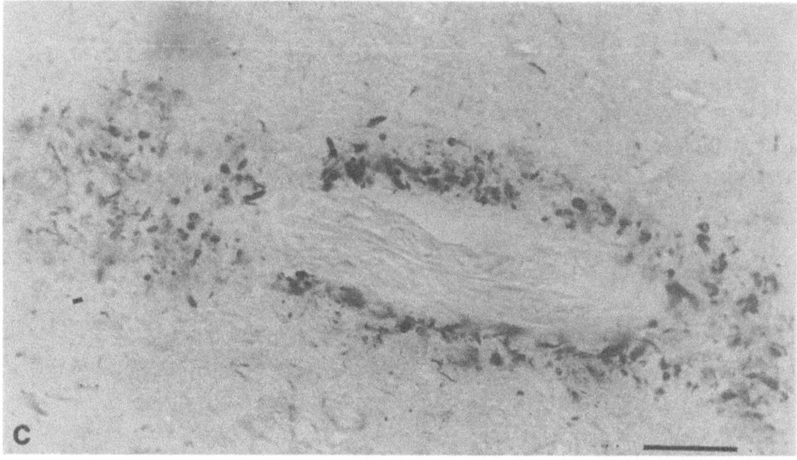

Fig. 3

pathological blood vessels, leading to the degeneration of neurites and then to the formation of PHF. PHF are probably the neuronal response to a variety of cellular insults, as observed for example in dementia pugilistica. PHF/AA were only observed in three cases of senile dementia of the Alzheimer type (SDAT) who had died after a long illness, and these cases showed severe congophilic angiopathy. The formation of PHF/AA, which is not a constant feature of Alzheimer's disease, might be due to the extensive amyloid deposits in vessel walls which probably impair the blood-brain barrier and provoke poisoning of the neighboring nerve parenchyma. Therefore, PHF/AA are probably a late consequence of the angiopathic amyloidosis and are certainly not a mechanism that explains the early events of Alzheimer's disease.

However, the determination of the pathogenesis of such lesions is interesting because they may explain, on a larger scale, the formation of SP. Since Miyakawa et al. (1982) demonstrated that SP contain a pathological capillary in their center, it may be possible that the mechanisms responsible for SP formation are identical to those leading to the formation of the PHF/AA lesions. Therefore, our observation seems to favor the hypothesis formulated by many authors that in Alzheimer's disease, a toxic material brought from blood vessels (possibly abnormal protein due to a gene defect) might lead first to the deposit of amyloid fibrils in the vicinity of the vessel and then to the degeneration of surrounding neurites, later provoking the aggregation of tau proteins in PHF. The random poisoning of neurites at the periphery of a vessel would show that Alzheimer's disease is a multitransmitter disease. It remains to be seen if the "geographic association of plaques with capillaries" is statistically significant or is no more than a geographic coincidence (Masters 1986).

The Degradation of PHF

There is great variety in the morphology of NFT and SP in the brain of patients with Alzheimer's disease probably due to the transformation of the lesions during the course of the illness. In order to understand the path of degradation of these lesions, we have observed the lesions with the double labeling technique (anti-PHF and thioflavine staining)

Observation of NFT and SP

NFT, which mainly contain bundles of PHF, were analyzed in detail. Simultaneous labeling with anti-PHF and thioflavine-S staining revealed different populations of globular tangles: strongly thioflavine-stained neurons were weakly labeled by anti-PHF whereas weakly thioflavine-stained perikaryons were intensely immunolabeled. The heterogeneity in the labeling was also observed in the same NFT. As a matter of fact, we frequently found, in the same degenerating pyramidal cell, areas of NFT that were weakly thioflavine stained and strongly immunolabeled and vice versa. The ghost tangles, which are the dissociated remnants of NFT (Rasool et al. 1984) were often only thioflavine stained (Fig. 4).

SP were also observed with the double labeling. Thioflavine staining revealed the strongly fluorescent core of SP surrounded by fluorescent wisps. This core was not immunolabeled by the anti-PHF but was encircled by a ring of mixed, strongly and weakly labeled neurites (Fig. 4).

PHF Bundles Progressively Acquire the Physical Properties of the Amyloid Substance

During degeneration of the neurons, NFT gradually seemed to lose their immunoreactivity and to acquire amyloid tinctorial properties. The same results were obtained by Wolozin et al. (1986). This transformation of NFT would explain the heterogeneity of their biochemical and tinctorial properties.

Thus, during this transformation, the spatial protein conformation of tangles could be modified and antigenic sites could be hidden (Allsop et al. 1986). In the same way, soluble NFT would become insoluble (Iqbal et al. 1984; Hussey et al. 1987), and NFT would be degraded both by a binding of ubiquitin to stimulate endogeneous proteo-lysis (Mori et al. 1987) and by anarchic phosphorylation (Bancher et al. 1987). Thus, NFT become eosinophilic and are penetrated by astrocytic processes (Probst et al. 1982; Yamaguchi et al. 1987). As early as 1927, Divry suggested that intracellular amyloid would become extracellular. All these observations support the hypothesis that PHF bundles in NFT and in degenerating neurites of SP progressively become a strongly thioflavine-stained amyloid material. They also acquire specific epitopes that are different from those of native tau proteins.

However, if bundles of PHF become an amyloid substance, this substance differs from the amyloid substance observed in the plaque core and in the vessel walls, which was never immunolabeled with the anti-PHF. Thus, at least two amyloid substances are present in the Alzheimer-affected cortex: the PHF-derived amyloid substance and the amyloid substance constituted by protein A4 which is a fragment of a 70-kd membrane receptor (Wong et al. 1985; Kang et al. 1987).

Conclusion

Using different techniques – immunoblotting, immunolabeling at optical and ultra-structural levels, and thioflavine staining – we have analyzed the different steps involved in the formation and transformation of PHF. The study of PHF is essentially concerned with two types of lesions: NFT and SP where bundles of PHF are found. However, it seems clear from the literature that NFT and SP have their own etiopathology. There is a near consensus that SP are the more specific lesions of Alzheimer's disease and that they are more likely to be the primum movens of the illness than NFT (Bartus, 1986).

The results presented here provide new data on three different aspects of the formation and transformation of PHF:

1. Tau proteins, the major antigenic components of PHF, are essentially distributed in the areas of normal cortical gray matter where PHF-containing lesions are found in Alzheimer's disease. These results suggest that tau proteins are not axonal proteins and that the aggregation of tau proteins in cell bodies is not directly related to a defect of axonal transport.

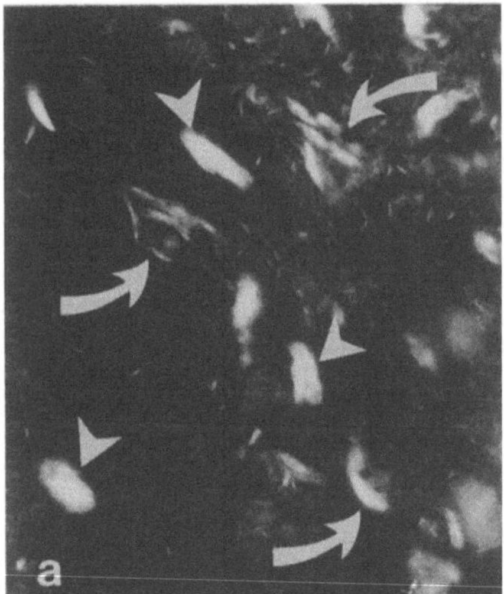 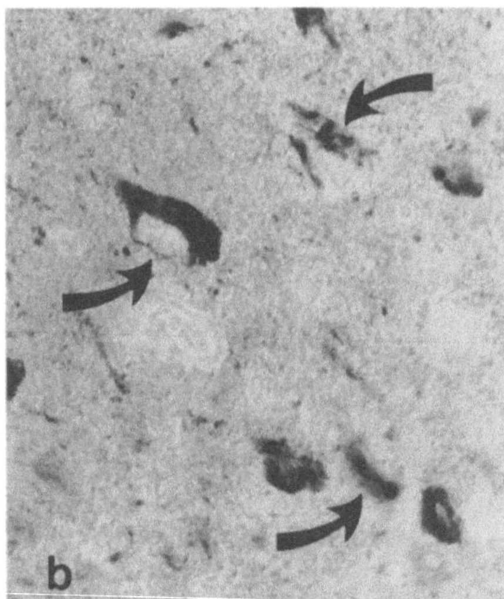

Fig. 4a–f. Double staining of paraffin sections by thioflavine and anti-PHF (Bar, 20 μm). **a, b** NFT on a paraffin section of Alzheimer-affected hippocampus observed with *a* fluorescence optics and *b* bright-field optics. Note the tangles simultaneously stained with anti-PHF and thioflavine (*arrows*) and tangles exclusively stained with thioflavine (*arrowheads*). **c, d** NFT on a paraffin section of Alzheimer-affected hippocampus observed with **c** fluorescence optics and **d** simultaneously with fluorescence optics and low-intensity bright-field optics. Immunostained tangles look different from thioflavine-stained ghost tangles. **e, f** SP on a paraffin section of Alzheimer-affected temporal cortex observed with *e* fluorescence optics and *f* bright-field optics. The strongly fluorescent central plaque core is not immunoreactive whereas surrounding neurites are simultaneously thioflavine stained and immunolabeled After the indirect peroxidase method as described by Delacourte and Défossez, 1986a), sections were incubated for 8 min in a 1% thioflavine-S aqueous solution and washed in 80% alcohol

2. The observation of PHF/AA lesions seems to favor the hypothesis that Alzheimer lesions, particularly SP, result from vascular poisoning, with PHF formation being a secondary phenomenon.
3. The transformation of PHF into an amyloid substance which is not immunologically related to the amyloid deposits of SP core and vessel walls suggests that different amyloid deposits of different origin are present in the brain affected by Alzheimer's disease.

Since Alzheimer's disease seems to be a poisoning of nerve endings of certain neuronal systems corresponding to the association cortex, it is now important to investigate the cause of the selective poisoning or of the vulnerability which leads to a morphological degeneration. Biochemical analysis of the different amyloid substances found in the brain will probably provide a rapid answer.

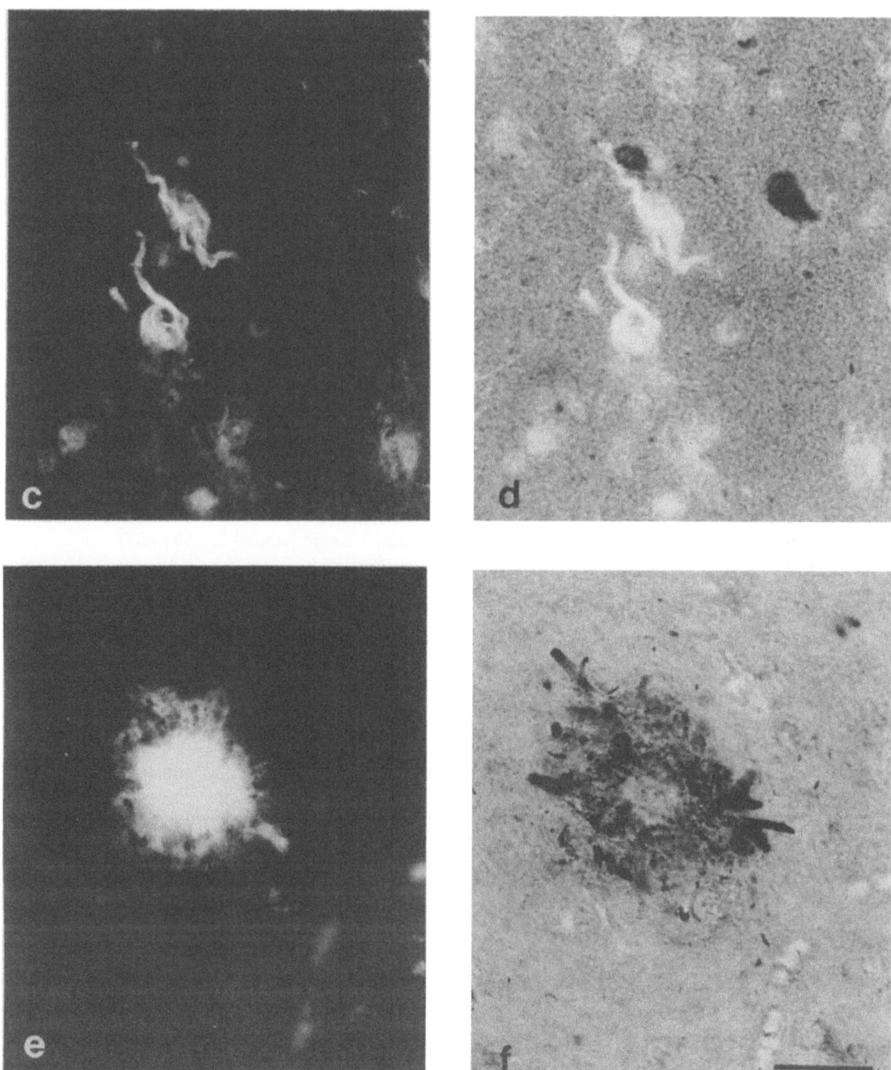

Fig. 4

References

Allsop D, Landon M, Kidd M, Lowe JJ, Reynolds GP, Gardner A (1986) Monoclonal antibodies raised against a subsequence of senile plaque core protein react with plaque cores, plaque periphery and cerebrovascular amyloid in Alzheimer's disease. Neurosci Lett 68: 252–256

Bancher C, Lassmann H, Budka H, Grundke-Iqbal I, Iqbal K, Wiche G, Seitelberger F, Wisniewski HM (1987) Neurofibrillary tangles in Alzheimer's disease and progressive supranuclear palsy: antigenic similarities and differences. Acta Neuropathol 74: 39–46

Bartus RT ed (1986) Controversial topics on Alzheimer's disease: intersecting crossroads. Neurobiol Aging 7: nb 6

Beauvillain JC, Tramu G, Garaud JC (1984) Coexistence of subtances related to enkephalin and somatostatin in granules of the guinea pig median eminence: demonstration by use of Colloidal gold immunocyto-chemical methods. Brain Res 301: 989–992

Binder LI, Frankfurter A, Rebhun LI (1985) The distribution of tau in the mammalian central nervous system. J Cell Biol 101: 1371–1378

Brion JP, Passareiro H, Nunez J, Flament-Durand J (1985) Immunological detection of tau protein in neurofibrillary tangles of Alzheimer's disease. Arch Biol 95: 229–235

Défossez A, Persuy P, Tramu G, Delacourte A (1986) Les lésions histologiques de la maladie d'Alzheimer. L'Encéphale 12: 161–168

Défossez A, El Hachimi K, Beauvillain JC, Perre J, Delacourte A, Foncin JF (1987) Etude immunocytochimique à l'échelle ultrastructurale des dégénérescences neurofibrillaires dans la maladie d'Alzheimer. CR Acad Sci [III] 304: 217–222

Delacourte A, Défossez A (1986a) Alzheimer's disease: tau proteins, the promoting factors of microtubule assembly, are major components of paired helical filaments. J Neurol Sci 76: 173–186

Delacourte A, Défossez A (1986b) Demonstration of a specific immunoreactivity of an antiserum against paired helical filaments and microtubule-associated proteins tau. In: Bès A et al. (eds) Senile dementia: early detection. Libbey Eurotext, Paris, pp 574–578

Delacourte A, Défossez A, Persuy P, Peers MC (1987) Observation of morphological relationships between angiopathic blood vessels and degenerative neurites in Alzheimer's disease. Virchows Arch [A] 411: 199–204

Divry PJ (1927) Etude histochimique des plaques séniles. J Belge Neurol 27: 643–657

Foncin JF, El Hachimi KH (1986) Neurofibrillary degeneration in Alzheimer's disease: a discussion with a contribution to aluminium pathology in man. In: Bès A et al. (eds) Senile dementias 86 – early detection. Libbey Eurotext, Paris, pp 191–201

Gambetti P, Perry G, Autilio-Gambetti L (1986) Paired helical filaments: Do they contain neurofilament epitopes? Neurobiol Aging 7: 451–452

Glenner GG (1983) Alzheimer's disease: multiple cerebral amyloidosis. In: Katzman R (ed) Biological aspects of Alzheimer's disease, Banbury report 15. Cold Spring Harbor, New York, pp 137–143

Grundke-Iqbal I, Iqbal K, Tung YC, Quinlan M, Wisniewski HM, Binder LI (1986a) Abnormal phosphorylation of the MAP tau in Alzheimer cytoskeletal pathology. Proc Natl Acad Sci USA 83: 4913–4917

Grundke-Iqbal I, Iqbal K, Quinlan M, Tung YC, Zaidi MS, Wisniewski HM (1986b) Microtubule-associated protein tau, a component of Alzheimer paired helical filaments. J Biol Chem 261: 6084–6088

Guiroy DC, Miyazaki M, Multhaup G, Fisher P, Garruto RM, Beyreuther K, Masters CL, Simms G, Gibbs CJ, Gajdusek C (1987) Amyloid of neurofibrillary tangles of Guamanian parkinsonism-dementia and Alzheimer disease share identical amino acid sequence. Proc Natl Acad Sci USA 84: 2073–2077

Hussey S, Yates CM, Christie JE, Elton RA, Gordon A (1987) Alzheimer-type dementia and Down's syndrome – solubility of neurofibrillary tangles is related to duration of dementia. J Neurol Neurosurg Psychiatry 50: 823

Ihara Y, Nukina N, Miura R, Ogawara M (1986) Phosphorylated tau protein is integrated into paired helical filaments in Alzheimer's disease. J Biochem (Tokyo) 99: 1807–1810

Iqbal K, Zaidi T, Thompson CH, Merz PA, Wisniewski HM (1984) Alzheimer paired helical filaments: bulk isolation, solubility and protein composition. Acta Neuropathol (Berl) 62: 167–177

Kang J, Lemaire HG, Unterbeck A, Salbaum JM, Masters CL, Grzeschik KH, Multhaup G, Beyreuther G, Muller-Hill B (1987) The precursor of Alzheimer's disease amyloid A4 protein resembles a cell-surface receptor. Nature 325: 733–736

Kidd M (1963) Paired helical filaments in electron microscopy of Alzheimer's disease. Nature 197: 192–193

Kosik KS, Joachim CL, Selkoe DJ (1986) Microtubule-associated protein tau is a major antigenic component of paired helical filaments in Alzheimer disease. Proc Natl Acad Sci USA 83: 4044–4048

Ksiezak-Reding H, Dickson DW, Davies P, Yen SH (1987) Recognition of tau epitopes by anti-neurofilament antibodies that bind to Alzheimer neurofibrillary tangles. Proc Natl Acad Sci USA 87: 3410–3414

Littauer UZ, Giveon D, Thierauf M, Ginzburg I, Ponstingl H (1986) Common and distinct tubulin binding sites for microtubule-associated proteins. Proc Natl Acad Sci USA 83: 7162–7166

Masters CL (1986) Disordered innervation of cerebral vasculature as a cause of Alzheimer's disease plaques and tangles. Neurobiol Aging 7: 516

Masters CL, Multhaup G, Simms G, Pottgiesser J, Martins RN, Beyreuther K (1985) Neuronal origin of a cerebral amyloid: neurofibrillary tangles of Alzheimer's disease contain the same protein as the amyloid of plaque cores and blood vessels. EMBO J 4: 2757–2763

Miller CCJ, Eagles PAM, Brion JP, Downes MJ, Calvert R, Flament-Durand J, Chin TK, Haugh M, Kahn J, Probst TA, Ulrich J, Anderton BH (1986) Alzheimer's paired helical filaments share epitopes with neurofilament side-arms. EMBO J 5: 269–276

Miyakawa T, Shimoji A, Kuramoto R, Higuchi Y (1982) The relationship between senile plaques and cerebral blood vessels in Alzheimer's disease and senile dementia. Morphological mechanism of senile plaque production. Virchows Arch [B] 40: 121–129

Miyakawa T, Katsuragi S, Watanabe K, Shimoji A, Ikeuchi Y (1986) Ultrastructural studies of amyloid fibrils and senile plaques in human brain. Acta Neuropathol (Berl) 70: 202–208

Mori H, Kondo J, Ihara Y (1987) Ubiquitin is a component of paired helical filaments in Alzheimer's disease. Science 235: 1641–1644

Nukina N, Ihara Y (1986) One of the antigenic determinants of PHF is related to tau protein. J Biochem (Tokyo) 99: 1541–1544

Nukina N, Kosik KS, Selkoe DJ (1987) Recognition of anti-PHF by monoclonal neurofilament antibodies is due to crossreaction with tau proteins. Proc Natl Acad Sci USA 87: 3415–3420

Persuy P, Defossez A, Delacourte A, Tramu G, Bouchez B, Arnott G (1985) Anti-PHF antibodies: an immunohistochemical marker of the lesions of the Alzheimer's disease. Virchows Arch [A] 407: 13–23

Probst A, Ulrich J, Heitz PU (1982) Senile dementia of Alzheimer type: astroglial reaction to extracellular neurofibrillary tangles in the hippocampus. Acta Neuropathol (Berl) 57: 75–79

Rasool CG, Abraham C, Anderton BH, Haugh M, Kahn J, Selkoe DJ (1984) Alzheimer's disease: immunoreactivity of neurofibrillary tangles with anti-neurofilament and anti paired helical filament antibodies. Brain Res 310: 249–260

Selkoe DJ, (1986) Altered structural proteins in plaques and tangles: what do they tell us about the biology of Alzheimer's disease. Neurobiol Aging 7: 425–432

Selkoe DJ, Bell DS, Podlisny MB, Price DL, Cork LC (1987) Conservation of brain amyloid proteins in aged mammals and humans with Alzheimer's disease. Science 235: 873–877

Wisniewski HM, Merz GS (1983) Neuritic and amyloid plaques in senile dementia of the Alzheimer type. In: Katzman R (ed) Biological aspects of Alzheimer's disease, Banbury report 15. Cold Spring Harbor, New York, pp 145–153

Wolozin BL, Pruchniki A, Dickson DW, Davies P (1986) A neuronal antigen in the brains of Alzheimer patients. Science 232: 648–650

Wong CW, Quaranta V, Glenner GG (1985) Neuritic plaques and cerebrovascular amyloid in Alzheimer disease are antigenically related. Proc Natl Acad Sci USA 82: 8729–8732

Wood JG, Mirra SS, Pollock NJ, Binder LI (1986) Neurofibrillary tangles of Alzheimer disease share antigenic determinants with the axonal microtubule-associated protein tau. Proc Natl Acad Sci USA 83: 4040–4043

Yamaguchi H, Morimatsu M, Hirai S, Takahashi K (1987) Alzheimer's neurofibrillary tangles are penetrated by astroglial processes and appear eosinophilic in their final stages. Acta Neuropathol (Berl) 72: 214–217

Yen SH, Dickson DW, Crowe A, Butler M, Shelanski ML (1987) Alzheimer's neurofibrillary tangles contain unique epitopes and epitopes in common with the heat-stable microtubule associated proteins tau and MAP2. Am J Pathol 126: 81–91

Amyloidosis in the Genesis of Alzheimer's Disease

G. G. Glenner

Summary

Based upon the precedent of previous studies on amyloidosis, the cerebrovascular amyloid fibrils from Alzheimer's disease and Down's syndrome have been isolated and amino acid sequencing performed. This revealed a unique 4.2-kd protein, designated the β-protein. This protein has also been identified as the amyloid fibril protein of "senile" plaques and the gene encoding for it resides on chromosome 21. The proximal source of amyloid β-protein is probably an immunoreactive serum protein. Characterization of this serum protein may lead to a specific diagnostic test for Alzheimer's disease.

Introduction

Dating from the time of Virchow, the mystery of the nature and origin of "amyloid" has attracted research workers from numerous diverse disciplines. Amyloid deposits are now known to be associated with more disease processes than any other condition, with the possible exception of cancer. The use by Virchow (1855) of the botanical term "amyloid" (starch or cellulose-like) for a human disease process tended to obscure its nature and pathogenesis. The definition and nature of the tissue deposits known as amyloid led to the assumption, and proof in 1970, that "amyloid" is a generic term describing the deposition of a twisted β-pleated sheet fibrillar protein, identified histologically by its Congo red staining and subsequent optical polarization properties (Glenner 1980).

Once it was demonstrated that unique fibrillar components comprised over 90% of amyloid deposits, efforts were made to obtain homogenous concentrates of these proteinaceous fibrils in order to subject them to analyses that would explain their chemical nature. These hopes were not fulfilled until methods were devised for making a solution of the amyloid fibrils with denaturing solvents that permitted fractionation of their constituent protein or proteins (Glenner et al. 1970). Analyses of these purified amyloid-fibril proteins led directly to the definition of major classes of amyloid-fibril proteins of unanticipated chemical diversity and, in some cases, to the identification of the origin of the fibril protein precursor. A wide variety of proteins (Glenner 1980, 1981), the amyloid disease complex (Glenner 1986a), have been defined as capable of being formed into amyloid fibrils since a group of immunoglobulin light polypeptide chains (AL) was first definitively described (Glenner et al. 1970, 1971b). Isotypes of the serum proteins prealbumin and serum amyloid-A (SAA) are capable of forming systemic amyloid fibrils of Familial amyloidosis (Portuguese variant) (AFp) and amyloid-A protein (AA) types, respectively, while local deposits of a precalcitonin protein form the amyloid deposits in medullary carcinoma of the thyroid (AE_t).

One major mechanism of systemic amyloid fibril deposition is proteolysis, as initially demonstrated in vitro (Glenner et al. 1971a). However, it was apparent that not all members of a class of potentially amyloid-forming precursor proteins, e.g., free immunoglobulin light chains, could be transformed into amyloid fibrils by proteolysis. The concept of the amyloidogenic protein evolved as a result, signifying that only specific precursor proteins (isotypes) could be converted in vivo to amyloid fibrils (e.g., the lambda VI light chain). A major pathogenetic mechanism for systemic amyloidosis was therefore thought to be proteolysis of an amyloidogenic precursor within phagocytic cells, e.g., macrophages, endothelial or synovium-lining cells (Glenner 1980).

Other physicochemical mechanisms could be invoked to explain localized amyloid deposits, e.g., AE_t (Glenner et al. 1974). In one category iatrogenic manipulation causes systemic concentration and subsequent precipitation of an amyloidogenic protein, β_2-microglobulin (Gorevic et al. 1986). Differences in amyloid deposit localization in the systemic disorders can be attributed to both the difference in lysosomal enzyme complement of phagocytic cells from site to site (Pitt 1975) and to the chemical nature of the substrate. Thus, peripheral but not central nervous system deposition in vascular walls is seen in AL and AA types of amyloidosis while only cerebral amyloidosis is observed in Alzheimer's disease (Glenner 1983) and Icelandic hereditary cerebral hemorrhage with amyloidosis (HCHWA) (Cohen et al. 1983).

Cerebrovascular Amyloidosis

The amino acid sequencing of an amyloid fibril protein (Glenner and Wong 1984a) in cerebrovascular amyloidosis (congophilic angiopathy) led to an approach to the unraveling of the nature of the cerebral amyloid fibrils (and perhaps the pathogenesis) of Alzheimer's disease. The basic premise, based on precedents from other amyloid diseases, was that amyloidosis is not a benign or irrelevant lesion when it affects the vasculature of the cerebrum. The resulting theory (Glenner 1979) suggested for the first time that an abnormal serum protein (gene product) was formed into amyloid fibrils by vascular cell (probably endothelial) enzyme proteolysis of an abnormal serum precursor. The chronic vascular mural deposition of fibrils leads to an incompetent blood-brain barrier and to chronic seepage of proteins (abnormal and/or neurotoxic) into the neuropil to eventuate in the formation of plaques and tangles, the former by proteolysis of an amyloidogenic (abnormal) precursor and the latter by perturbation of the intracellular neuronal milieu (Glenner et al. 1974) as the result of neurotoxic serum protein blockade of neuronal receptors. Since this was a testable theory, the first requisite was to determine whether cerebrovascular amyloidosis was a concomitant of plaques and tangles in the vast majority of patients diagnosed as having Alzheimer's disease.

Earlier studies reported that all cases of cerebrovascular amyloidosis were associated with either plaques or dementia (Pantelakis 1954; Surbeck 1961). Conversely, there were scattered reports (Corsellis 1984) of cerebrovascular amyloidosis occurring in "normal" aged brains. However, the only two conditions other than Alzheimer's disease consistently having significant cerebrovascular amyloid deposits are hereditary cerebral hemorrhage with amyloidosis (HCHWA) (Cohen et al. 1983) and adult Down's syndrome (Glenner 1983). A survey (Glenner 1983; Glenner et al. 1981; G.G. Glenner, unpublished data) of 700 brains of clinically and pathologically diagnosed Alzheimer's disease patients revealed that 92% had associated cerebrovascular amyloidosis. Age-matched controls, including those with hypertension, in which plaques and tangles were uniformly absent, failed to show cerebrovascular amyloidosis at autopsy (Glenner et al. 1981), whilst in demented individuals, no patients had cerebrovascular amyloidosis unassociated with senile plaques and tangles.

The isolation of the cerebrovascular amyloid fibers from Alzheimer's disease and adult (over 40 years old) Down's syndrome individuals was then initiated (Glenner and Wong 1984a, b). Histologic examination revealed a continuum of amyloid deposition from the leptomeningeal to the intracortical vessels (Glenner et al. 1981). The assumption was made that the chemical nature of the intracortical vascular deposits was the same as that of the leptomeningeal vessels. To avoid contamination by congophilic material from cerebral plaques and tangles, only the amyloid-laden vessels of the leptomeninges were utilized for amyloid fibril isolation. The leptomeningeal amyloid deposits were isolated, the fibrils were concentrated to homogeneity and denatured in 6 M guanidine hydrochloride, and the major amyloid fibril protein was purified by high-performance liquid chromatography. Amino acid sequence analysis to position 24 (Glenner and Wong 1984a, b) and subsequently to position 28 (Wong et al. 1985) revealed this to be a unique 4.2-kd protein, previously unsequenced, and homologous (one amino acid substitution difference) to that isolated from the leptomeningeal amyloid-laden vessels in Down's syndrome adults. This 4.2-kd protein was designated β-protein (Glenner and Wong 1984a). Polyclonal antibodies raised to the synthetic 1–10 peptide of β-protein coupled through its C-terminal amino acid to keyhole-limpet hemocyanin revealed, under stringent immunohistochemical control, localization of the antibodies not only to leptomeningeal and intracortical vascular amyloid deposits but also to plaques in both Alzheimer's disease and adult Down's syndrome (Glenner et al. 1984; Wong et al. 1985). No localization to neurofibrillary tangles could be observed, nor were amyloidotic vessels in HCHWA reactive, as would be expected, since the amyloid fibril protein of HCHWA is an isotype of a cystatin C (gamma trace) protein. A recent electron microscopic study employing the β-protein antibodies and an immunogold technique has localized these antibodies to the amyloid fibrils of the vessels (Ikeda et al. 1987). This study, in addition to the chemical evidence, supports the contention that β-protein is an integral component of the amyloid fibrils.

Plaque Amyloid Fibril Protein

The amino acid sequencing of the amyloid core of senile plaques obtained from cases of Alzheimer's disease and Down's syndrome individuals was attempted by Masters et al. (1985a). They obtained an inseparable series of at least four polypeptides by HPLC fractionation which had progressive deletions of their N-terminal amino acids (N-terminal heterogeneity). They ordered these peptides according to the amino acid sequence of β-protein and found homology with it, except for discrepancies in position 11 (Glu for Gln). An amino acid variation of 50% from that reported by Masters et al. was subsequently found by us (Wong et al. 1985) in the terminal four amino acids of the 28 amino acid β-protein sequence, i.e., in position 27 (Ser for Asn) and 28 (Ala for Lys). It is doubtful whether, without the 24 amino acid sequence of the cerebrovascular amyloid β-protein reported earlier (Glenner and Wong 1984a), these polypeptides could have been ordered into sequence, since at each cycle at least four amino acids would have been detected.

Masters et al. (1985a) also failed to demonstrate whether their protein was the major protein isolated and/or whether it might be due to cerebrovascular amyloid contamination. They also apparently assumed that all plaques were at the same stage of N-terminal peptide cleavage, that the number of polypeptides (four) with N-terminal heterogeneity represented a temporal sequence, and that they could date by their number the age of the plaque deposits relative to those in other lesion sites, e. g., cerebrovascular amyloid deposits. Whether the fact that pepsin digestion used in Masters and coworkers' purification scheme contributed to the N-terminal heterogeneity of their proteins is presently unknown. However, the finding of normally occurring N-terminal heterogeneity in amyloid fibril proteins purified in the absence of proteolytic enzymes is not unusual (Benditt et al. 1971) and is presumably due to endogenous proteolytic limit digests. Masters et al. (1985b) assumed that there was no heterogeneity at the N-terminal sequence of the cerebrovascular amyloid fibril protein whereas at least two different N-terminal polypeptides have since been described (Glenner 1986b).

Masters et al. dated the plaque amyloid protein as occurring earlier than that in the vessels on the basis of the increased N-terminal heterogeneity. Even assuming that the extent of N-terminal heterogeneity would date plaque deposits, the argument is negated by the probability that the amyloid is in a different stage of deposition (diffuse to compact) from plaque to plaque and, therefore, some plaques may have a complete β-protein amino acid sequence and others a varying one, but individually uniform extent of N-terminal heterogeneity. The assumption also fails in view of the likelihood that the cellular complement of enzymes responsible for cerebrovascular proteolysis (endothelial) is probably different from the one responsible for intracerebral proteolysis (microglial).

Neurofibrillary Tangles

Total solubilization of the paired helical filaments of the neurofibrillary tangles has yet to be convincingly realized, though numerous proteins have been ascribed to be the paired helical filament protein both by chemical extraction (Masters et al. 1985b; Grundke-Igbal et al. 1986) and by immunohistochemical methods (Wood et al. 1986; Anderton et al. 1982). Masters et al. (1985b) attempted the extraction of the paired helical filament protein and obtained seven inseparable polypeptides which they ordered to be homologous with β-protein. The arguments for such an amino acid sequence interpretation without prior alignment to the β-protein sequence are even less plausible with seven simultaneous amino acid signals than they were for the four of the senile plaque. The possibility that the β-protein sequence of the tangles results from contaminating amyloidotic cerebral vessels has been suggested (Selkoe et al. 1986). The temporal sequence of cerebral fibril deposition from neurofibrillary tangles to produce amyloid fibrils in plaques and subsequently in vessels, as suggested by Masters et al. (1985b), appears unlikely, especially in view of the lack of physiologic rationale to explain how neuronal fibrillary material is deposited in leptomeningeal vessel walls.

These same authors, employing the synthetic peptides 1–11 and 11–23 of β-protein coupled by unknown means to keyhole-limpet hemocyanin described immuno-histochemical localization of antibodies to peptide 1–11 to tangles and those to peptide 11–23 to plaques and vessel amyloid. No inhibition studies or other confirmatory evidence of reaction specificity were described. Masters et al.'s immunohistochemical localization of β-protein peptide antibodies to neurofibrillary tangles has thus far not been confirmed (Wong et al. 1985; Allsop et al. 1986; Selkoe et al. 1986). Poly- and monoclonal antibodies to peptide 1–10 and polyclonal antibodies to peptide 21–28 react in my experience, only with the plaques and vascular amyloid of Alzheimer's disease and of adult Down's syndrome (G.G. Glenner, unpublished observations). However, as previously indicated (Wong et al. 1985), this lack of reactivity of the neurofibrillary tangles may be due to steric factors. Ultrastructural localization of β-protein antibodies to the amyloid fibrils of both cerebral vessels and senile plaques has now been achieved by an immunogold method (Ikeda et al. 1987), providing further evidence that β-protein is an integral component of these amyloid fibrils.

A β-pleated sheet structure for the paired helical filaments of the neurofibrillary tangles has been suggested, based on their tinctorial and optical properties after Congo red staining (Glenner et al. 1974) and X-ray crystallographic studies (Kirshner et al. 1985). If this is confirmed, the speculated causative association of aluminum with these structures (Perl and Brody 1980) will be explainable as the result of selective absorption or liganding of aluminum ions to the side chains of the β-structure (Glenner 1977). Thus, in such a situation the accumulation of aluminum would be an epiphenomenon and not causative in the formation of the tangles. A classic example of this is calcium binding to amyloid fibers and the subsequent calcium-dependent liganding of the Amyloid P component protein to all amyloid exposed to this serum protein (Glenner 1980).

Discussion

What we now know is that a protein antigenically related to β-protein is present in senile plaques and cerebrovascular amyloid deposits. Since a β-protein-related substance is found in both plaques and cerebrovascular amyloid, this finding markedly increases the likelihood that cerebrovascular amyloid deposition is related to Alzheimer's disease. As previously noted, this suggests that the formation of neuritic plaques is the result of compromises of the blood-brain barrier (Wong et al. 1985). Since the amyloid fibril protein of the senile plaques is less soluble than that of the vessels (Roher et al. 1986), this could signify that the precursor of the fibril protein of the plaque is a larger fragment of its putative β-serum precursor or is adducted to other organic or inorganic compounds.

The significance of proteolysis cannot be underestimated in the pathogenesis of Alzheimer's disease. Recent evidence from molecular genetic studies (Goldgaber et al. 1987) indicates that the gene product is an approximately 150-kd protein and that increased gene dosage occurs in Alzheimer's disease and Down's syndrome (Delabar et al. 1987). The immunochemically related putative β-protein precursor in serum is approximately 60 kd (see below). The senile plaque amyloid fibril protein is about 6 kd and the cerebral vascular fibril protein is 4.2 kd. Thus it appears that progressive proteolysis leads to the conversion of the nascent gene product to the amyloid fibril. What is of major significance is the nature of the proteolytic enzymes(s) that converts the putative serum precursor to the fiber. Since, in Alzheimer's disease and in HCHWA, amyloid deposition occurs only in cerebral vessels and not in peripheral vessels, it must be assumed that the enzyme complement hydrolyzing the β-protein precursor of Alzheimer's disease (and the cystatin C variant of HCHWA) in endothelial cells differs between the periphery and central nervous system. In addition, as the β-protein precursor leaks through the amyloid-disrupted blood-brain barrier of the cerebral vessels, a different complement of proteolytic enzymes (possibly microglial) acts on it to form the amyloid fibers of senile plaques. The variance in size of the protein of the plaque amyloid fibrils (6 kd) and the vascular protein (4.2 kd) strongly suggests that the fibrils in these two sites result from processing by different enzyme complements.

The presence of plaques, tangles, and cerebrovascular amyloid in virtually all cases of adult Down's syndrome is one of great interest in the potential solution of the nature and pathogenesis of Alzheimer's disease. Since the β-protein is found in identical lesions in both disorders, this should also be the case for the putative abnormal serum precursor and the abnormal gene which synthesizes it (Glenner 1983; Glenner and Wong 1984b; Wong et al. 1985). It might be suggested that if a serum precursor of the amyloid fibrils were found in all Down's syndrome individuals, both under and over the age of 40, and the same serum protein were found in pathologically diagnosed Alzheimer's disease patients, then this protein would be a marker for those individuals destined to develop Alzheimer's disease (of particular value for familial genetic counseling). That an abnormal serum precursor to the β-protein exists is based on the fact that, when systemic vascular amyloid deposits are found in other amyloidotic conditions, they derive from an abnormal serum protein (Glenner 1980; Terry et al. 1973; Dwulet and Benson 1984). As previously noted, the identification of such a protein should lead to a specific diagnostic serum or genomic test for Alzheimer's disease (Glenner and Wong 1984b; Wong et al. 1985). In view of the homologous amino acid sequence of β-protein in Alzheimer's disease and Down's syndrome, it was predicted that the amyloid β-protein gene would be detected on chromosome 21 (Glenner 1983; Glenner and Wong 1984b). This has now been confirmed (Goldgaber et al. 1987).

On Western blots in Alzheimer's disease serum, we have identified three 60–64 kd proteins antigenically reactive to monoclonal antibodies to peptide 1–10 of β-protein (Glenner 1986b) and are in the process of isolating these proteins in order to characterize them chemically. Based on the concept of amyloidogenic proteins and precedent, e. g., the prealbumin 30 variant (Dwulet and Benson 1984), it is possible that polymorphism will be expressed for genomic β-protein precursor in Alzheimer's disease. This should manifest itself in a normal β-protein precursor in normal individuals, and in a normal and one or more isotypic proteins (one of which is amyloidogenic) in Alzheimer's disease and in Down's syndrome. This polymorphism may lead to a specific diagnostic serum test for Alzheimer's disease.

Acknowledgments. We wish to express our appreciation to Karen Rasmussen for technical assistance, and to Dennis Olshefsky for peptide synthesis. Alzheimer's disease tissues were obtained from the University of California at San Diego National Alzheimer's Disease Brain Bank.

This research was supported by grants from the National Institute of Health, AG-05683, and from the California State Department of Health Services, 84-84559

References

Allsop D, Landon M, Kidd M, Lowe JS, Reynolds GP, Gardner A (1986) Monoclonal antibodies raised against a subsequence of senile plaque core protein react with plaque cores, plaque periphery and cerebrovascular amyloid in Alzheimer's disease. Neurosci Lett 68: 252–256

Anderton BH, Breinburg D, Downes MJ, Green PJ, Tomlinson BE, Ulrich J, Wood JN, Kahn J (1982) Monoclonal antibodies show that neurofibrillary tangles and neurofilaments share antigenic determinants. Nature 298: 84–86

Benditt EP, Eriksen N, Hermodson MA, Ericsson LH (1971) The major proteins of human and monkey amyloid substance: common properties including unusual N-terminal amino acid sequences. FEBS 19: 169–173

Cohen DE, Feiner H, Jensson O, Frangione B (1983) Amyloid fibril in hereditary cerebral hemorrhage with amyloidosis (HCHWA) is related to the gastroenteropancreatic neuroendocrine protein, gamma trace. J Exp Med 158: 623–628

Corsellis JAN (1984) Aging and the dementias. In: Blackwood W, Corsellis JAN (eds) Greenfield's neuropathology, 4th ed. Year Book Medical Publishers, Chicago, pp 951–1025

Delabar JM, Goldgaber D, Lamour Y, Nicole A, Huret JL, Grouchy J, Brown P, Grajdusek DC, Sinet PM (1987) β amyloid gene duplication in Alzheimer's disease and karyotypically normal Down's syndrome. Science 235: 1390–1392

Dwulet FE, Benson MD (1984) Primary structure of an amyloid prealbumin and its plasma precursor in a heredofamilial polyneuropathy of Swedish origin. Proc Natl Acad Sci USA 81: 694–698

Glenner GG (1977) Factor X deficiency and systemic amyloidosis (editorial). N Engl J Med 297: 108

Glenner GG (1979) Congophilic microangiopathy in the pathogenesis of Alzheimer's syndrome (presenile dementia). Med Hypotheses 5: 1231–1236

Glenner GG (1980) Amyloid deposits and amyloidosis: the β-fibrilloses (medical progress report). N Engl J Med 302: 1283–1292, 1333–1343

Glenner GG (1981) Amyloidosis: the hereditary disorders including Alzheimer's disease (editorial). J Lab Clin Med 98: 807–810

Glenner GG (1983) Alzheimer's disease: multiple cerebral amyloidosis. In: Katzman R (ed) Biological Aspects of Alzheimer's disease, Banbury report 15, Cold Spring Harbor symposium. Cold Spring Harbor Laboratory, pp 137–144

Glenner GG (1986a) Amyloid research as a paradigm for Alzheimer's disease. In: Glenner G, Osserman E (eds) Amyloidosis. Plenum, New York, pp 693–702

Glenner GG (1986b) Beta protein, a possible marker for Alzheimer's disease. In: Glenner GG, Wurtman RJ (eds) Advancing frontiers in Alzheimer's disease. Austin, University of Texas Press, pp 125–136

Glenner GG, Wong CW (1984a) Alzheimer's disease: initial report of the purification and characterization of a novel cerebrovascular amyloid protein. Bichem Biophys Res Commun 120: 885–890

Glenner GG, Wong CW (1984b) Alzheimer's disease and Down's syndrome: sharing of a unique cerebrovascular amyloid fibril protein. Biochem Biophys Res Commun 122: 1131–1135

Glenner GG, Harbaugh J, Ohms JI, Harada M, Cuatrecasas P (1970) An amyloid protein: the amino terminal variable fragment of an immunoglobulin light chain. Biochem Biophys Res Commun 41: 1287–1289

Glenner GG, Ein D, Eanes ED, Bladen HA, Terry W, Page D (1971a) The creation of amyloid fibril from Bence Jones in vitro. Science 174: 712–714

Glenner GG, Terry W, Harada M, Isersky C, Page D (1971b) Amyloid fibril proteins: proof of homology with immunoglobulin light chains by sequence analyses. Science 172: 1150–1151

Glenner GG, Eanes ED, Bladen HA, Linke RP, Termine JD (1974) β-Pleated sheet fibrils: a comparison of native amyloid with synthetic protein fibrils. J Histochem Cytochem 22: 1141–1158

Glenner GG, Henry JH, Fujihara S (1981) Congophilic angiopathy in the pathogenesis of Alzheimer's degeneration. Ann Pathol 1: 120–129

Glenner GG, Wong CW, Quaranta V, Eanes ED (1984) The amyloid deposits in Alzheimer's disease: their nature and pathogenesis. Appl Pathol 83: 7908–7912

Goldgaber D, Lerman MI, McBride OW, Saffiotti U, Gajdusek DC (1987) Characterization and chromosomal localization of a cDNA encoding brain amyloid of Alzheimer's disease. Science 23: 877–880

Gorevic PD, Munoz PC, Casey TT, DiRaimondo CR, Stone WJ, Prelli FC, Rodrigues MM, Poulik MD, Frangione B (1986) Polymerization of intact β2-microglobulin in tissue causes amyloidosis in patients on chronic hemodialysis. Proc Natl Acad Sci USA 83: 7908–7912

Grundke-Iqbal I, Iqbal K, Quinlan M, Tung Y, Zaidi MS, Wisniewski HK (1986) Microtubule-associated protein tau: a component of Alzheimer paired helical filaments. J Biol Chem 261: 6084–6089

Ikeda S, Wong CW, Allsop D, Landon M, Kidd M, Glenner GG (1987) Immunogold labeling of cerebrovascular and neuritic plaque amyloid fibrils in Alzheimer's disease with an anti β-protein monoclonal antibody. Lab Invest 57: 446–449

Kirschner DA, Abraham CA, Selkoe DJ (1985) X-ray diffraction from intraneuronal paired helical filaments and extraneuronal amyloid fibers in Alzheimer disease indicates cross-β conformation. Proc Natl Acad Sci USA 87: 503–512

Masters CL, Simms G, Weinman NA, Multhaup G, McDonald BL, Beyreuther K (1985a) Amyloid plaque core protein in Alzheimer disease and Down syndrome. Proc Natl Acad Sci USA 82: 4245–4249

Masters CL, Multhaup G, Simms G, Pottgiesser J, Martins RN, Beyreuther K (1985b) Neuronal origin of a cerebral amyloid: neurofibrillary tangles of Alzheimer's disease contain the same protein as the amyloid of plaque cores and blood vessels. EMBO J 4: 2757–2763

Pantelakis S (1954) Un type particulier d'angiopathie sénile du système nerveux central: l'angiopathie congophile. Topographie et fréquence. Monatsschr Psychiatr Neurol 128: 219–256

Perl DP, Brody AR (1980) Alzheimer's disease: x-ray spectrometric evidence of aluminium accumulation in neurofibrillary tangle-bearing neurons. Science 208: 297–299

Pitt D (1975) Lysosomes and cell function. Longman, London, p 165

Roher A, Wolfe D, Palutke M, KuKuruga D (1986) Purification, ultrastructure, and chemical analysis of Alzheimer disease amyloid plaque core protein. Proc Natl Acad Sci USA 83: 2662–2666

Selkoe DJ, Abraham CR, Podlisny MB, Duffy LK (1986) Isolation of low-molecular-weight proteins from amyloid plaque fibers in Alzheimer's disease. J Neurochem 46: 1820–1834

Surbeck EB (1961) L'angiopathie dyshorique (Morel) de l'écorce cérébrale: étude anatomoclinique et statistique: aspect génétique. Acta Neuropathol (Berl) 1: 168–197

Terry WD, Page DL, Kimura S, Isobe T, Osserman EF, Glenner GG (1973) Structural identity of Bence Jones and amyloid fibril proteins in a patient with plasma cell dyscrasia and amyloidosis. J Clin Invest 52: 1276–1281

Virchow R (1855) Zur Cellulose-Frage. Virchows Arch [A] 8: 140–144

Wong CW, Quaranta WV, Glenner GG (1985) Neuritic plaques and cerebrovascular amyloid in Alzheimer disease are antigenically related. Proc Natl Acad Sci USA 82: 8729–8732

Wood JG, Mirra SS, Pollock NJ, Binder LI (1986) Neurofibrillary tangles of Alzheimer disease share antigenic determinants with the axonal microtubule-associated protein tau (τ). Proc Natl Acad Sci USA 83: 4040–4043

Protein Chemical and Molecular Biological Studies of Amyloid Precursor Proteins in Alzheimer's Disease

D. J. Selkoe

Summary

Available information about the classical structural lesions of Alzheimer's disease (AD) provides a complex picture of paired helical filament (PHF) and amyloid fibril composition. In the case of the intraneuronal fibers, the microtubule-associated phosphoprotein tau is an antigenic constituent of the PHF and related straight filaments. It is not yet clear to what extent MAP2 and neurofilament proteins also contribute to PHF. Ubiquitin and possibly other neuronal proteins are present in addition to tau. Neurofibrillary degeneration appears to involve an alteration and insolubilization of certain microtubule-associated proteins together with other constituents that remain to be clarified. Whether this process, which occurs in a number of unrelated neurofibrillary disorders, depends solely on abnormal postranslational processing of cytoskeletal proteins and/or involves changes in transcriptional or translation control of the expression of neuronal proteins remains to be seen.

The weight of current evidence suggests that the brain amyloid filaments that accumulate in AD, Down's syndrome and normal brain aging but are absent in other neurofibrillary tangle-forming disorders are distinct from PHFs. A major component of amyloid fibrils found both in senile plaque cores and in meningeal and cortical blood vessels is a low molecular weight hydrophobic protein (the β-protein) with a previously unknown sequence. Recent studies from several laboratories indicate that the gene encoding this amyloid protein is localized to chromosome 21. This observation provides a direct link to the virtually invariable occurrence of senile plaques and vascular amyloid in Down's syndrome. However, our studies do not confirm reports of elevated gene dosage of the β-protein in AD patients. The finding of amyloid deposits in normal aged humans and aged mammals that are immunochemically highly similar to AD amyloid suggests that a mechanism for accelerated amyloid deposition in selective brain regions occurs in patients with AD. The precise cellular origin of the amyloid precursor protein that gives rise to the filaments found in cerebral vessels and neuropil is not yet clear. The initial identification of amyloid-associated proteins (e. g., α-1 antichymotrypsin) raises the possibility that proteins distinct from the β-protein could be involved in the cleavage and local processing of the β-protein precursor.

Introduction

In contrast to numerous brain degenerative diseases in which neuronal loss is unaccompanied by any characteristic structural change in adjacent neurons that have not yet died, neuronal attrition in Alzheimer's disease (AD) is associated with marked changes in many remaining cells and in the neuropil. Neuritic (senile) plaques, amyloid angiopathy and neurofibrillary tangles (NFTs) represent the principal structural alterations of the brain in presenile and senile dementia of the Alzheimer type. These types of lesions are also found in much smaller numbers and with restricted topographical distribution in the brains of neurologically normal individuals after the seventh decade. Tangles, plaques, and other structural changes found in AD brain tissue [amyloid angiopathy of cerebral and meningeal vessels, granulovacuolar degeneration of hippocampal neurons, lipofuscin (LF) deposition in neurons and glia] are, therefore, qualitatively indistinguishable from the lesions that accompany normal brain aging but are quantitatively much increased in AD. As a result, knowledge about the formation of fibrous changes in AD should provide insight into certain mechanisms of human brain aging in general. The principal objective of current work in several laboratories is to characterize the molecular mechanism of paired helical filament (PHF) and amyloid fibril formation and to establish what role this process may play in accelerated dysfunction and death of neurons during aging and in AD.

Despite doubts expressed over the years about the utility of analyzing the plaques and tangles, it appears increasingly likely that molecular studies of these fibrous lesions can provide important insights into the pathogenesis and perhaps even the etiology of progressive cortical degeneration in AD. It should be emphasized at the outset that NFTs, with their characteristic PHFs, are a much less specific lesion for AD than is the neuritic plaque with its associated amyloid deposit. NFTs occur in a wide variety of etiologically diverse brain disorders, including metabolic, viral, traumatic, and toxic insults. In contrast, the amyloid-bearing neuritic plaques which occur invariably in AD, are otherwise found only in aged normal individuals and in patients with trisomy 21 (Down's syndrome). Thus, studies of the genesis of neuritic plaques and the role of amyloidogenic proteins in this process appear more likely to provide clues about seminal events in AD than does the analysis of NFTs.

The Neurofibrillary Tangle and its Paired Helical Filaments

The accumulation of abnormal cytoplasmic fibers in neuronal cell bodies and in the neurites of senile plaques has been statistically correlated with the principal features of AD, including degree of dementia, extent of neuronal loss in hippocampus, and degree of deficiency of cortical cholinergic function. NFTs are non-membrane-bound masses of abnormal fibers found within the perikaryal cytoplasm of neurons. Numerous electron microscopic studies have concluded that the majority of fibers in these tangles have the appearance of tightly adherent pairs of helical filaments (PHFs). These organelles have a maximum width of about 20 nm and a half-periodicity of roughly 80 nm (Kidd 1963; Terry 1963; Wisniewski et al. 1976). Many of the abnormal neurites (both axonal terminals and dendrites) making up the periphery of the senile plaque contain PHF (Gonatas et al. 1967). In recent years it has been increasingly reported that bundles of straight (nonhelical) filaments of approximately 15–20 nm width may also be found in neurons in AD-affected brains and may coexist with PHFs in the same cells (Metuzals et al. 1981; Selkoe 1984; Shiboyama and Kitoh 1978; Yagashita et al. 1981).

In my experience, certain cases of clinically and light microscopically typical AD have been associated with perikaryal and neuritic filaments that are almost entirely straight, with few if any visible PHFs (D. J. Selkoe, unpublished observations). Such cases may show ready disaggregation of the tangles in gentle or harsh solvents; this fact may explain the observation of Iqbal and colleagues that certain AD cases have a high percentage of "soluble" tangles (Iqbal et al. 1984). It is not yet clear whether the individual straight filaments comprising such tangles are solubilized into subunit polypeptides or are only disaggregated and therefore no longer microscopically visible after solvent treatment; certainly, some straight filaments can be recovered in sodium dodecyl sulfate (SDS)-insoluble pellets from such brains.

In addition to recognizing bundles containing PHFs and/or abnormal straight filaments in the neurites of senile plaques, antibodies to such fibers (see below) can detect the relevant antigens in fine cortical neurites that are widely dispersed in the cerebral cortex and not organized into neuritic plaques. This immunochemical evidence of a more widespread alteration of neurites is in accordance with early electron microscopic studies of the AD cerebral cortex (Kidd 1963; Terry 1963). Thus the histopathological concept of AD as a "plaque and tangle disease" is a simplification. In fact, a more widespread and complex disruption of the neuritic architecture of the cerebral cortex is observed.

NFT also occur in another morphological form; i. e., bundles of abnormal filaments lacking associated neuronal structure and apparently lying free in the extracellular neuropil. Such presumed extracellular tangles, referred to as ghost tangles or tombstones, are particularly prevalent in certain brain regions that are prone to marked NFT formation, e.g., entorhinal, cortex, parahippocampal gyrus, and nucleus basalis. It is generally believed that these structures represent the fibrous residua of the once-intraneuronal tangles. One may further speculate that parts or all of these extracellular fibrous masses are slowly catabolized and disappear, since long-surviving cases of AD often display only moderate numbers of ghost tangles in addition to classical intraneuronal NFT. Alzheimer himself, and other early students of AD, described the putative transition of neuronal tangles into extracellular fibrous masses. This morphological change is accompanied by an immunochemical transition in which the amount of PHF-reactive antigens is substantially lower in extracellular than intraneuronal tangles.

The identity and origin of the constituent proteins of the PHF has become a matter of considerable interest. The first reported protein chemical studies of cortical fractions containing NFTs or partially purified PHFs found enrichment of a polypeptide of molecular weight 50000 daltons in such fractions (Iqbal et al. 1974). This protein was felt to be a constituent of the PHF and was referred to as the paired helical filament protein (PHFP) (Iqbal et al. 1974). Immunocytochemical studies with antisera raised against gel-purified PHFP (Grundke-Iqbal et al. 1979a) and against a partially purified human brain microtubule preparation (Grundke-Iqbal et al. 1979b) showed staining of Alzheimer NFTs in tissue sections. These and other immunochemical studies by Iqbal and colleagues led to the conclusion that antigens other than tubulin, present in microtubule fractions from the normal brain, are shared with PHFs. The precise identification and characterization of these antigens were not further described.

Studies by Yen and coworkers (1981) confirmed that polyclonal antisera to crude human microtubule preparations stained ≈ 40% of the NFTs in AD-affected cortex as well as the neurites of the senile plaque. These authors as well as Eng et al. (1980) found that antibodies to tubulin itself did not stain the tangles. Numerous other immunocytochemical studies (reviewed in Selkoe 1986) showed that many polyclonal and monoclonal antibodies against neurofilaments do not cross-react with NFTs and senile plaque neurites, whereas certain neurofilament antibodies do. The results of these various efforts suggested a complex antigenic composition of the abnormal fibers, including portions of neurofilament – and microtubule-associated proteins.

Following the discovery (Selkoe et al. 1982) of the marked insolubility of most PHFs in strong detergents and solvents (e.g., SDS, β-mercaptoethanol, urea), it became apparent that two related problems were hampering the characterization of PHFs: their insolubility and the consequent difficulty in purifying them and isolating their subunit proteins. To date, a method for the rigorous, high-grade purification of PHFs from brain tissue has not been found, although methods that lead to considerable enrichment of the filaments are available (Ihara et al. 1983; Iqbal et al. 1984; Selkoe and Abraham 1986). As a result, investigators have been forced to continue to use immunocytochemistry to delineate further some of the proteins contributing to PHFs.

Both polyclonal (Ihara et al. 1983) and monoclonal (Selkoe et al. 1985; Wang et al. 1984; Yen et al. 1985) antibodies raised directly against partially purified PHF have generally failed to recognize normal cellular structures or specific fibrous proteins in adult human brain tissue. This paradox has been resolved in part by the discovery by several groups that brain fractions highly enriched in the microtubule-associated phosphoprotein tau react strongly with PHF polyclonal antibodies and also with some monoclonal PHF antibodies (Brion et al. 1985; Grundke-Iqbal et al. 1986; Kosik et al. 1986; Nukina and Ihara 1986; Wood et al. 1986). Conversely, these same studies showed that antibodies raised against normal tau prepared from various mammalian brains almost always recognize NFTs and altered neurites in AD and normal aged cortex. These and other results have led to the widely accepted conclusion that tau, which is actually a heterogeneous family of phosphoproteins ranging in molecular weight from 50000 – 66000 daltons is a principal antigenic constituent of PHF and also of related straight filaments that are seen in Pick's disease, progressive supranuclear palsy (PSP), and certain other neurofibrillary diseases. However, the extent to which tau contributes to total PHF composition is unknown, since stoichiometry is precluded by the insolubility and lack of purity of the fibers. It is now known that other neuronal proteins, distinct from tau, contribute to or are at least closely associated with PHF. For example, extensive absorption of polyclonal PHF antibodies with normal tau still leaves the antisera capable of recognizing NFT and neurites in AD-affected cortex. This result suggests that polyclonal antisera to PHF contain antibodies directed against highly altered forms of tau or against distinct proteins. One such non-tau component of PHF has recently been identified by Mori and colleagues (1987). These investigators used a monoclonal PHF antibody and mixtures of peptides cleaved proteolytically from PHF-enriched or normal brain fractions to identify the protein ubiquitin as an additional component of the pathological fibers. Subsequent immunocytochemical studies with antibodies to native ubiquitin have confirmed the association of ubiquitin not only with AD tangles but also with Pick's bodies, Lewy bodies in the brain in Parkinson's disease, and tangles in PSP (Perry et al. 1987; Terry 1987). Among its numerous functions, ubiquitin is known to bind to altered or short-lived cellular proteins prior to their ATP-dependent proteolysis. Whether this mechanism occurs unsuccessfully in AD neurons remains unknown.

Mounting evidence indicates that the tau proteins associated with PHFs have properties distinct from those of normal tau. For example, tau epitopes in PHFs are resistant to postmortem effects and formalin fixation, in contrast to tau in normal axons, which is often difficult to demonstrate in sections of fixed human brain. Also, the tau found in fibrillary lesions is present in a highly insoluble form, in contrast to the marked solubility of tau prepared from normal mammalian brain.

The fact that virtually all tau antibodies tested to date react with tangles and neurites in AD-affected brain has led to a reexamination (Ksiezak-Reding et al. 1987; Nukina et al. 1987) of the rather small subset of neurofilament monoclonal antibodies that also recognize these lesions. A number of these antibodies have now been shown to recognize phosphorylated forms of tau. In vitro dephosphorylation of tau or neurofilament proteins decreases or abolishes their reactivity with such neurofilament antibodies. Similarly, dephosphorylation of tangles in brain sections also removes their immunoreactivity. Conversely, certain antibodies against nonphosphorylated neurofilament proteins that do not recognize AD tangles also do not react with tau (Nukina et al. 1987). Due to these recent studies there is now much stronger evidence implicating tau as an antigenic component of PHF than there is implicating neurofilament proteins. Nonetheless, further studies are needed to demonstrate whether neurofilament proteins and another microtubule-associated protein, MAP2 (Kosik et al. 1984) are constituents of the fibers.

Although the possibility of covalent cross-linking in PHF exists, an alternative mechanism for explaining the insolubility of PHF derives from recent X-ray diffraction studies. Kirschner and colleagues (1986) have carried out X-ray diffraction analysis of isolated PHF and senile plaque amyloid cores. Using considerably enriched but not fully purified PHF preparations, we observed characteristic $\approx$ 4.76-Å and $\approx$ 10.6-Å reflections consistent with a macromolecule containing cross-β-pleated sheet conformation. This finding appears to confirm the long-held hypothesis that, like other amyloids, the intraneuronal PHFs in AD contain a β-pleated sheet structure. Analyses of highly purified senile plaque core amyloid gave similar patterns (Kirschner et al. 1986). The β-pleated sheet conformation of PHF and amyloid fibers could explain, at least in part, their high degree of insolubility. However, the lack of quantitative solubilization of PHF and amyloid cores by concentrated guanidine HCl differs from the behavior of most amyloid fibers in nonneural organs and suggests an even greater degree of insolubility in the fibers of AD.

On the basis of comparative studies of pathological fibers occurring in a variety of unrelated neurodegenerative disorders, it can be said that the various conclusions about PHF summarized above apply equally to the NFTs in a number of human neurological conditions (see, e.g., Joachim et al. 1987b). Thus, there is no current evidence that AD involves a special or unique neuronal cytoskeletal reorganization not seen in other human brain disorders. More likely, progressive protein alteration and formation of abnormal filamentous structures in neuronal cytoplasm may represent a somewhat nonspecific response of certain classes of human neurons to a variety of insults. To date, no specific antigenic or other biochemical characteristics of PHFbearing neurons in AD have been identified to distinguish them from the tangle-bearing neurons found in normal aging, the Guam Parkinson-dementia complex, and other degenerative diseases.

The Amyloid Deposits of Neuritic Plaques and Cerebral Microvessels

In addition to the intraneuronal fibrous changes just described, AD-affected brain tissue displays abundant extracellular deposits of abnormal filaments that are found in the cores of senile plaques, in small bundles in the cortical neuropil, and in the walls of certain leptomeningeal and cortical blood vessels (congophilic angiopathy). Like the NFTs, these fibrous extracellular deposits show characteristic green birefringence under polarized light after staining with the dye Congo red and are fluorescent after staining with thioflavine. Electron microscopy (EM) demonstrates that the filaments comprising these deposits are generally in the range of 6–10 nm in diameter (mean ≈ 8 nm) and are unpaired. Their fine structure is distinct from that of the intraneuronal PHF and straight filaments.

In order to separate senile plaque amyloid from other constituents of AD-affected cortex and to characterize it, we used a novel strategy, fluorescence-activated cell sorting (FACS), to isolate intact amyloid cores in an aqueous suspension (Selkoe et al. 1986a). The discrete, roughly spherical nature of the cores and the fact that their size (6–20 μm in maximal diameter) is similar to blood cells that are routinely separated by flow cytometry led us to this approach. Initial core fractions were prepared by centrifuging SDS-extracted homogenates of AD-affected cortex at low speed, allowing quantitative pelleting of the cores while many LF granules, NFT, and small particles remained in the supernatant. The suspension was then sieved and separated on sucrose density gradients. Gradient interfaces that were particularly enriched in cores were subjected to FACS. Using fluorescence and light-scattering (size) discriminants, unlabeled cores were separated from most autofluorescent LF granules by an initial FACS. The cores were then rhodamine-labeled with an antiserum raised against partially purified amyloid cores and were separated from remaining contaminants by a second FACS. Bright-field fluorescence and polarization microscopy of the final fraction revealed highly purified, intact amyloid cores. EM showed that the cores were virtually free of contaminants except for occasional aggregates of LF. From particle counting, the final fractions consisted of ≥ 90% amyloid cores, the remainder being LF and rare capillary fragments.

Amino acid analyses of such FACS-purified core fractions demonstrated a composition that includes approximately 50% nonpolar residues with abundant glycine and no proline (Selkoe and Abraham 1985; Selkoe et al. 1986a). When we obtained this composition for purified cores, it was apparent that it was highly similar to the composition of the meningovascular amyloid protein (the β-protein) reported by Glenner and Wong (1984). Moreover, antibodies we raised against a hydrophobic low molecular weight (400 – 700 daltons) protein released by formic acid or guanidine thiocyanate from our FACS-purified cores stained both plaque cores and amyloid in meningeal and cortical microvessels (Selkoe et al. 1986a). This result was also obtained by Wong et al. (1985) using antibodies not to the native amyloid protein but to a synthetic β-amyloid peptide.

Despite this immunochemical cross-reaction, we observed differences between plaque and vascular amyloid in the AD-affected brain. Firstly, compacted amyloid cores are insoluble in 6 M guanidine HCl (Masters et al. 1985b; Selkoe et al. 1986a), the reagent used by Glenner and Wong to solubilize and isolate the meningovascular β-amyloid protein. Secondly, neither we (Selkoe et al. 1986a) nor others (Bobin et al. 1987; Gorevic et al. 1986) have been able to sequence the core-derived low molecular weight protein, although we are readily able to obtain an unambiguous β-protein sequence (through residue 30) from meningovascular amyloid prepared by an SDS-isolation method (Joachim et al. 1987a), confirming the seminal sequence data provided by Glenner and Wong (1984). Thus, the compacted amyloid deposits found in the centers of neuritic plaques, while related by antigenicity and amino acid composition to microvascular amyloid, appear to have a blocked or buried N-terminus and are insoluble in guanidine HCl. These properties suggest a further processing (in the case of the plaque amyloid) of a common precursor protein.

It appears, therefore, that the amyloid fibers in plaques and vessels in AD are principally composed of a low molecular weight, hydrophobic fragment of the β-protein that readily aggregates to form polymers. The presence of similar proteins in PHF-enriched fractions may be due to contaminating amyloid filaments in these fractions rather than to the PHFs. Virtually all available immunochemical evidence from numerous laboratories suggests that the amyloid filaments found extracellularly in AD-affected brain tissue are not composed of the same neuronal proteins (including tau and ubiquitin) that comprise the PHF. Furthermore, PHFs occur abundantly in several human neurologic diseases in which one sees no amyloid deposition or neuritic plaque formation whatsoever. Also, aged primates and other mammals develop microvascular and senile plaque amyloid deposits that cross-react with several AD amyloid antibodies (including those to the β-peptide); however, these animals have no PHFs or NFTs and the neurites of their plaques are not reactive with tau and PHF-antibodies (Selkoe et al. 1987a). In both AD and normal aging, amyloid filaments that are immunochemically and protein-chemically highly similar to those in senile plaque cores occur in the walls of meningeal arteries outside of the brain, a location that makes a direct neuronal origin less likely. A recent report (B. Frangione, personal communication) that cerebrovascular deposits of the β-protein can occur in middle-aged humans without formation of discrete plaque cores and with no NFT underscores the latter point. The obtaining of partial sequences of the β-protein from plaque core-enriched (Masters et al. 1985b) or NFT-enriched (Masters et al. 1985a) AD brain fractions may be due to the presence in such fractions of contaminating vascular amyloid filaments, which can readily be sequenced. However, despite these various considerations, further careful work will be needed to determine whether the PHFs contain a central protein filament that is composed of the same β-polypeptide as the extraneuronal amyloid filaments; such a possibility cannot be excluded at present.

Information about the partial amino acid sequence of the amyloid β-protein led to the use of oligonucleotides to clone cDNAs for this protein from brain expression libraries (Goldgaber et al. 1987; Kang et al. 1987; Robakis et al. 1987; Tanzi et al. 1987). As a result, the β-amyloid gene was localized to the long arm of human chromosome 21, approximately in the region 21q21. Among the first developments that arose from these findings was the report that three patients with apparently sporadic AD had a 50% increased dosage of the beta amyloid gene on chromosome

21, similar to the elevation of dosage found in patients with trisomy 21 (Delabar et al. 1987). This finding was interpreted by the authors to indicate a microduplication, presumably occurring during meiosis, of a subsegment of chromosome 21 in the region of the β-amyloid gene. Because of the potential importance of this observation for understanding the pathogenesis of AD and for diagnosis of the disease, we undertook a larger study of 36 patients, 14 with clinically diagnosed AD, ten with trisomy 21, and 12 aged control subjects (Podlisny et al. 1987). We carried out densitometric analyses of Southern blots probed with a cDNA for the β-protein to determine the relative dosage of this gene in genomic DNA from these 36 individuals. Whereas the ten patients with trisomy 21 showed the expected 1.5-fold increase in dosage of this gene, none of the 14 AD patients had a gene dosage higher than that of the normal controls. These results were statistically highly significant. Our results do not support recent reports that microduplication of a segment of chromosome 21 is the genetic basis of AD (Schweber et al. 1984; Delabar et al. 1987). Alternative mechanisms for the region-specific increase in β-protein deposition in the brain in AD patients compared with aged normal humans should be sought.

Although we were unable to document an increased gene dosage of the β-amyloid precursor protein in AD, we have recently used several antibodies to synthetic peptides from amyloid and nonamyloid regions of the precursor to detect an apparent increase in cross-reactive proteins in the cerebral cortex in AD (Selkoe et al. 1987). An antibody to β-peptide 1–28 recognizes a protein doublet at approximately 76000–83000 daltons at higher levels in the cortex of AD patients than in the normal cortex on Western blots. This enhanced protein also appears to be detected by two other amyloid protein antibodies, one to a threonine-rich synthetic peptide that is the N-terminal to the amyloid region and another to the 20 residues comprising the C-terminal of the precursor. An analysis of different regions of an AD-affected brain showed elevated amounts of these β-protein-reactive polypeptides in those regions that develop AD amyloid deposits, c. g., the neocortex from the four main lobes, the hippocampus, and even the striatum (in a case where abundant striatal plaques were found). In contrast, other regions of the same AD-affected brain (e. g., subcortical white matter, thalamus, pons, and cerebellum) that showed no amyloid plaque formation had the control levels of the 76000–83000 dalton immunoreactive doublet. Further characterization and purification of the immunoreactive proteins in cortical homogenates is under way. The results to date suggest that forms of the β-protein precursor found normally in the human brain are selectively increased in amount in the AD-affected brain, specifically in those regions prone to development of amyloid deposits (Selkoe et al. 1987 b). This finding suggests either enhanced expression of the precursor or alterations in its normal catabolism, apparently leading to local increases in the precursor and perhaps to abnormal proteolytic processing that could produce cleavage of the amyloidogenic region and subsequent filament formation.

Evidence that Protein(s) Distinct from the β-protein are Closely Associated with AD Amyloid

In characterizing several polyclonal antibodies to AD amyloid developed in our laboratory, we noted that certain antisera had very low or no reactivity with the amyloid β-protein. In particular, polyclonal antibodies raised against enriched fractions of intact amyloid filaments recognize the β-protein weakly but label amyloid deposits in plaque cores and vessels at very high titers. On the basis of such observations, we have tentatively categorized our amyloid antibodies into three groups, according to the immunogen used:

a) antisera to intact amyloid filaments,
b) antisera to the low molecular weight hydrophobic protein (β-protein) solubilized by formic acid from such amyloid filaments, and
c) antibodies to synthetic β-protein peptides. Groups b and c show reaction with the β-protein by dot immunoassay and on Western blots; in contrast, group – a antisera show weak or no reaction. All three groups of antisera stain amyloid deposits in AD-affected brain sections in a highly similar fashion.

Further elucidation of the distinct antigens recognized by these antibodies has emerged from attempts to identify normal plasma proteins that cross-react with amyloid. To date, only antibodies of group a, as described above, show unequivocal reaction with specific human plasma proteins (Selkoe et al. 1986b). The principal cross reactive plasma proteins identified by such antibodies are a doublet with approximate molecular weights of 88000 and 95000 daltons. We have partially purified these proteins from human plasma using ammonium sulfate fractionation and affinity gel chromatography. Tentative immunochemical identification of the 80000–95000 dalton bands suggests that they cross-react with antibodies to α-1 antichymotrypsin. This observation followed the work of Abraham et al. (1987) in which the same amyloid antiserum that identified these plasma proteins was used to screen human liver cDNA libraries. The three clones thus identified all encoded the serine protease inhibitor, α-1 antichymotrypsin. This hepatic-synthesized protein is abundantly present in normal plasma. The identification and cloning of this protein using antibodies to AD amyloid filaments raises the possibility that α-1 antichymotrypsin could play a role in the local processing of the β-amyloid precursor protein in the AD-affected brain. Several antibodies to α-1 antichymotrypsin immunolabel plaque and vascular amyloid deposits in sections of AD-affected brain, after the vigorous extraction of the plaque cores in SDS. However, it is also possible that the presence of this protein inhibitor represents nonspecific sticking of a serum protein to the hydrophobic amyloid filaments. Whether α-1 antichymotrypsin or other protease inhibitors and associated proteases play a role in the local processing of the amyloid β-precursors will be the subject of further study.

References

Abraham C, Selkoe DJ, Potter H (1987) A component of brain amyloid in Alzheimer's disease is the serine protease inhibitor, alpha-1 antichymotrypsin. Cell in press
Bobin SA, Currie JR, Chen M-C, Iqbal K, Miller DL, Styles JJ, Wisniewski HM (1987) Comparisons between the structures of cerebral vascular amyloid (CVA) and senile plaque core amyloid (SPCA) peptides found in Alzheimer's disease (abstract). Fed Proc Fed Am Soc Exp Biol 46: 2137
Brion JB, van Den Bosch de Aguilar P, Flament-Durand J (1985) In: Traber J, Gispens WH (eds); Advances in applied neurological science: senile dementia of the Alzheimer type. Springer, Berlin Heidelberg New York, pp 164–174

Eng LF, Forno LS, Bigbee JW, Forno KI (1986) Immunohistochemical localization of glial fibrillary acidic protein and tubulin in Alzheimer's disease brain biopsy material. In: Amaducci L, Davison AN, Antuono P (eds). Aging of the brain and dementia. Raven, New York, p 49

Delabar JM, Goldgaber D, Lamour Y, Nicole A, Huret JL, Grouchy J, Brown P, Grajdusek DC, Sinet PM (1987) β amyloid gene duplication in Alzheimer's disease and karyotypically normal Down's syndrome. Science 235: 1390–1392

Glenner GG, Wong CW (1984) Alzheimer's disease: initial report of the purification and characterization of a novel cerebrovascular amyloid protein. Biochem Biophys Res Commun 120: 885–890

Goldgaber D, Lerman MI, McBride OW, Saffiotti U, Gajdusek DC (1987) Characterization and chromosomal localization of a cDNA encoding brain amyloid of Alzheimer's disease. Science 235: 877–880

Gonatas NK, Anderson W, Evangelista I (1967) The contribution of altered synapses in the senile plaque: an electron microscopic study in Alzheimer's dementia. J Neuropathol Exp Neurol 26: 25–39

Gorevic P, Goni F, Pons-Estel B, Alvarez F, Peress R, Frangione B (1986) Isolation and partial characterization of neurofibrillary tangles and amyloid plaque core in Alzheimer's disease: immunohistological studies. J Neuropathol Exp Neurol 45: 647–664

Grundke-Iqbal I, Iqbal K, Quinlan M, Tung Y-C, Zaidi MS, Wiesniewski HM (1986) Microtubule-associated protein tau: a component of Alzheimer paired helical filaments. J Biol Chem 261: 6084–6089

Grundke-Iqbal I, Johnson AB, Terry RD, Wisniewski HM, Iqbal K (1979a) Alzheimer neurofibrillary tangles: antiserum and immunohistological staining. Ann Neurol 6: 532

Grundke-Iqbal I, Johnson AB, Wisniewski HM et al. (1976b) Evidence that Alzheimer neurofibrillary tangles originate from neurotubules. Lancet 1: 578

Ihara Y, Abraham C, Selkoe DJ (1983) Antibodies to paired helical filaments in Alzheimer's disease do not recognize normal brain proteins. Nature 304: 727–730

Iqbal K, Wisniewski HM, Shelanski ML et al. (1974) Protein changes in senile dementia. Brain Res 77: 337

Iqbal K, Zaidi T, Thompson CH, Merz PA, Wisniewski HM (1984) Alzheimer paired helical filaments: bulk isolation, solubility and protein composition. Acta Neuropathol (Berl) 32: 157–162

Joachim CL, Duffy LK, Selkoe DJ (1987a) Isolation and characterization of cerebrovascular amyloid (CVA) proteins in Alzheimer's disease (abstract). J Neuropathol Exp Neurol 46: 396

Joachim CL, Morris JH, Kosik KS, Selkoe DJ (1987b) Tau antisera recognize neurofibrillary tangles in a range of neurodegenerative disorders. Ann Neurol 22: 514–520

Kang J, Lemaire HG, Unterbeck A, Salbaum JM, Masters CL, Grzeschik K-H, Multhaup G, Beyreuther K, Muller-Hill B (1987) The precursor of Alzheimer's disease amyloid A4 protein resembles a cell-surface receptor. Nature 325: 733–736

Kidd M (1963) Paired helical filaments in electron microscopy of Alzheimer's disease. Nature 197: 192–193

Kirschner DA, Abraham CA, Selkoe DJ (1986) X-ray diffraction from intraneuronal paired helical filaments and extraneuronal amyloid fibers in Alzheimer disease indicates cross-β conformation. Proc Natl Acad Sci USA 83: 503–507

Kosik KS, Duffy LK, Dowling MM, Abraham C, McCluskey A, Selkoe DJ (1984) Microtubule-associated protein 2: monoclonal antibodies demonstrate the selective incorporation of certain epitopes into Alzheimer's neurofibrillary tangles. Proc Natl Acad Sci USA 81: 7941–7945

Kosik KS, Joachim CL, Selkoe DJ (1986) The microtubule-associated protein, tau, is a major antigenic component of paired helical filaments in Alzheimer's disease. Proc Natl Acad Sci USA 83: 4044–4048

Ksiezak-Reding H, Dickson DW, Davies P, Yen S-H (1987) Recognition of tau epitopes by anti-neurofilament antibodies that bind to Alzheimer neurofibrillary tangles. Proc Natl Acad Sci USA 84: 3410–3414

Masters CL, Multhaup G, Simms G, Pottgiesser J, Martins RN, Beyreuther K (1985a) Neuronal origin of a cerebral amyloid: neurofibrillary tangles of Alzheimer's disease contain the same protein as the amyloid of plaque cores and blood vessels. EMBO J 4: 2757–2763

Masters CL, Simms G, Weinman NA, Mvlthaup G, McDonald BL, Beyreuther K (1985b) Amyloid plaque protein in Alzheimer's disease and Down syndrome. Proc Natl Acad Sci USA 82: 4245–4249

86   D.J. Selkoe

Metuzals J, Montpetit V, Clapin DE (1981) Organization of the neurofilamentous network. Cell Tissue Res 214: 455–482

Mori H, Kondu J, Ihara Y (1987) Ubiquitin is a component of paired helical filaments in Alzheimer's disease. Science 235: 1641–1644

Nukina N, Ihara Y (1986) One of the antigenic determinants of paired helical filaments is related to tau protein. J Biochem (Tokyo) 99: 1541–1544

Nukina N, Kosik KS, Selkoe DJ (1987) Recognition of Alzheimer paired helical filaments by monoclonal antibodies is due to crossreaction with tau protein. Proc Natl Acad Sci USA 84: 3415–3419

Perry G, Friedman R, Shaw G, Chau V (1987) Ubiquitin is detected in neurofibrillary tangles and senile plaque neurites of Alzheimer disease brains. Proc Natl Acad Sci USA 84: 3033–3036

Podlisny MB, Lee G, Selkoe DJ (1987) Gene dosage of the β-amyloid precursor protein in Alzheimer's disease. Science 238: 669–671

Robakis NK, Wisniewski HM, Jenkins EC, Devine-Gage EA, Houck GE, Yao X-L, Ramakrishna N, Wolfe G, Silverman WP, Brown WT (1987) Chromosome 21q21 sublocalisation of gene encoding beta-amyloid peptide in cerebral vessels and neuritic (senile) plaques of people with Alzheimer disease and Down syndrome. Lancet 1: 385

Schweber M, Tuson C, Shiloh R, Ben-Neriah ZB (1987) Triplication of chromosome 21 material in Alzheimer's disease (abstract). Neurology 37 (Suppl 1): 222

Selkoe DJ (1984) The fibrous cytopathology of degenerating neurons in Alzheimer's disease: an ultrastructural reappraisal. Soc Neurosci Abstr 10: 813

Selkoe DJ (1986) Review: altered structural proteins in plaques and tangles: what do they tell us about the biology of Alzheimer's disease. Neurobiol Aging 7: 425–432

Selkoe DJ, Abraham C (1985) Plaque amyloid in Alzheimer's disease (AD): purification by flow cytometry and protein characterization (abstract). Neurology 35 (Suppl 1): 217

Selkoe DJ, Abraham C (1986) Isolation of paired helical filaments and amyloid fibers from human brain. In: Valee R (ed) Methods in enzymology, vol 134. Academic, New York, pp 388–404

Selkoe DJ, Ihara Y, Salazar FJ (1982) Alzheimer's disease: insolubility of partially purified helical filaments in sodium dodecyl sulfate and urea. Science 215: 1243–1245

Selkoe DJ, Abraham C, Rasool CG, McCluskey A, Duffy LK (1985) Production and characterization of monoclonal antibodies to Alzheimer paired helical filaments. Ann NY Acad Sci 455: 774–778

Selkoe DJ, Abraham CR, Podlisny MB, Duffy LK (1986a) Isolation of low-molecular-weight proteins from amyloid plaque fibers in Alzheimer's disease. J Neurochem 46: 1820–1834

Selkoe DJ, Galibert L, Podlisny M, Duffy LK (1986b) Normal human plasma proteins share antigenic determinants with CNS amyloid fibrils in Alzheimer's disease (AD). Soc Neurosci Abstr 12 (1): 35

Selkoe DJ, Bell DS, Podlisny MB, Price DL, Cork LC (1987a) Conservation of brain amyloid proteins in aged mammals and humans with Alzheimer's disease. Science 235: 873–877

Selkoe DJ, Saperstein A, Podlisny M, Duffy L (1987b) Antibodies to the amyloid β-protein detect an ~80 kDa brain protein at higher levels in Alzheimer than normal cortex but not in cerebellum (abstract). Soc Neurosci Abstr 316. 17

Shiboyama H, Kitoh J (1978) Electron microscopic structure of Alzheimer's neurofibrillary changes in a case of atypical senile dementia. Acta Neuropathol (Berl) 41: 229–234

Tanzi RE, Gusella JF, Watkins PC, Bruns GAP, St. George-Hyslop P, van Keuren ML, Patterson D, Paga S, Kurnit DM, Neve RL (1987) Amyloid β protein gene: cDNA mRNA distribution, and genetic linkage near the Alzheimer locus. Science 235: 880–884

Terry RD (1963) The fine structure of neurofibrillary tangles in Alzheimer's disease. J Neuropathol Exp Neurol 22: 629–642

Terry RD (1987) J Neuropath Exp Neurol submitted for publication

Wang GP, Grundke-Iqbal I, Kascsak RJ, Iqbal K, Wisniewski HM (1984) Alzheimer neurofibrillary tangles: monoclonal antibodies to inherent antigen(s). Acta Neuropathol (Berl) 62: 268–275

Wisniewski HM, Narong HK, Terry RD (1976) Neurofibrillary tangles of paired helical filaments. J Neurol Sci 27: 173–181

Wong CW, Quaranta V, Glenner GG (1985) Neuritic plaques and cerebrovascular amyloid in Alzheimer disease are antigenically related. Proc Natl Acad Sci USA 82: 8729–8732

Wood JG, Mirra SS, Pollock NJ, Binder LI (1986) Neurofibrillary tangles of Alzheimer's disease share antigenic determinants with the axonal microtubule-associated protein tau. Proc Natl Acad Sci USA 83: 4040–4043

Yagashita S, Itoh T, Nan W, Amano N (1981) Reappraisal of the fine structure of Alzheimer's neurofibrillary tangles. Acta Neuropathol (Berl) 54: 239–246
Yen SH, Gaskin F, Terry RD (1981) Immunocytochemical studies of neurofibrillary tangles. Am J Pathol 104: 77
Yen S-H, Crowe A, Dickson DW (1985) Monoclonal antibodies to Alzheimer's neurofibrillary tangles. I. Identification of polypeptides. Am J Pathol 120: 282–291

The Molecular Basis of Cerebral Amyloidosis in Alzheimer's Disease and the Unconventional Virus Diseases

C. L. Masters, R. Martins, G. Simms, B. Rumble, S. Fuller, L. Hutchinson, J. Beer, C. Hilbich, T. Dyrks, P. Fischer, A. Weidemann, U. Monning, G. Multhaup, M. Cramer, J. M. Salbaum, S. Wehr, and K. Beyreuther

Summary

The major protein subunit of the amyloid fibril in Alzheimer's disease is a small molecule of 42 residues (termed A4). It is derived from a larger precursor (PreA4), the gene for which is located on chromosome 21, in close proximity to the region involved in Down's syndrome. The predicted structure of PreA4 suggests that it is an integral membrane glycoprotein. Knowledge of the mechanisms by which PreA4 is degraded to A4 may contribute to a better understanding of the cause of Alzheimer's disease. Similarly, the amyloid fibril in the unconventional virus diseases is composed of the PrP molecule, which in turn is derived from a neuronal membrane glycoprotein. An understanding of the process by which the PrP molecule is converted into an amyloidogenic molecule may shed some light on the nature of the infectious unit.

Introduction

Although the proportion of the population with neuropathologically confirmed Alzheimer's disease (AD) increases exponentially with age (from 50 years onwards), AD is not an invariable component of the aging process. There are clearly genetic, epigenetic, and probably environmental factors which operate to induce the deposition of amyloid fibrils, which are the major structural anomaly in AD. The neuropathological diagnosis of AD has been difficult with conventional histologic techniques, but with more sensitive immunocytochemical screening procedures for the deposition of the A4 amyloid protein, a clearer picture is emerging (Davies et al. 1988).

The Molecular Basis of Cerebral Amyloidosis in AD

Pathognomonic amyloid deposition in AD is restricted to certain areas of the central nervous system and then occurs within two clearly definable compartments:

1. *Intracellular*. The fibrils polymerize to form neurofibrillary tangles (NFT) and "dystrophic" neurites composed of characteristic paired helical filaments (PHF) and single "straight" filaments. NFT occur in the soma of pyramidal cells and the

"dystrophic" neurites accumulate around the periphery of the extracellular amyloid deposits.

2. *Extracellular.* Amyloid fibrils first polymerize, then condense in a spherical fashion in the neuropil, and finally crystallize into an amyloid plaque core (APC). At the same time, and to a variable degree, the same molecular species polymerizes into amyloid fibrils around the walls of selected blood vessels to form an amyloid congophilic angiopathy (ACA).

The relationship of the amyloid plaque to the neuronal cell body is best illustrated by Probst's Golgi impregnation studies, which in turn highlight the Cajal's perspicaciousness when he described the neurites around the extracellular amyloid as "reactive."

The pioneering electron microscopic studies of Kidd, Terry, Wisniewski and Gonatos demonstrated the differences in the amyloid filaments comprising the NFT and APC, but we are still left with many unanswered questions on the fine structural analysis. All filaments, whether of intracellular or extracellular origin, appear to have a protofilamentous substructure with a paired or quadrupled helical arrangement.

The topographic distribution of the amyloid deposits (NFT, APC, and ACA) within the brain provide important information (Pearson et al. 1985; Rogers and Morrison 1985). In neocortical areas, NFT and APC have laminar distributions, with the NFT principally in layers III and V while the APC tend to be accentuated in layers II and III, and to a lesser degree in layers V and VI. The distribution of lesions neither correlates with any known neurotransmitter or neuropeptide system nor with any pattern of vascular distribution or vascular innervation. The lesions are more severe in association cortex and are less pronounced in the primary sensorimotor cortices, which are involved only in more severe cases. The only clear systematic distribution of lesions lies in the olfactory pathway, the hippocampus, the amygdala, and the basal forebrain nuclci.

Many authors have drawn attention to the autosomal dominantly inherited form of AD, familial AD (FAD) (Masters et al. 1981 a). It is probable that many cases of FAD go unrecognized and that the proportion of all cases of AD which are familial exceeds 50%.

The association of AD with Down's syndrome (DS) elucidates one of a number of possible pathways in the molecular pathogenesis of AD. Although conventional histology shows all DS patients have cerebral amyloid deposits by the age of 40, more sensitive immunocytochemical techniques now show that the amyloidogenic process begins much earlier.

Our strategy over the last few years has been to purify and biochemically characterize the amyloid deposits. A similar line of investigation was also pursued by groups in San Diego (Glenner), Nottingham (Kidd, Allsop, Landon), Boston (Selkoe), Detroit (Wolfe, Roher), New York (Frangione), Staten Island (Bobin, Iqbal, Wisniewski), and Tokyo (Ihara).

Glenner and Wong (1984a, b) were the first to purify and sequence the ACA material. We purified the APC from both AD and DS patients and showed that the principal subunit (termed A4) was a small protein (mass 4.5 kd) which was similar if not identical to Glenner's β-protein (Masters et al. 1985 a). The A4 protein had a great tendency to aggregate and form dimers, tetramers, and higher oligomeric species.

When we next purified an NFT preparation from AD and DS (Masters et al. 1985b), we found that the amyloid material in these preparations had a very similar biochemical profile to the APC preparations (similar in amino acid composition, SDS-gel electrophoresis, high-performance liquid gel chromatography, and N-terminal amino acid sequence). We concluded that the A4 subunit was also the principal component of the NFT. Many investigators could not accept this result because of the clear structural and immunochemical differences between NFT and APC or ACA. They attributed our results to the presence of contaminating APC or ACA within the NFT preparations (Gorevic et al. 1986). According, we next showed that the NFT in the Guam parkinsonism-amyotrophic lateral sclerosis complex (PD-ALS) was also composed of the A4 subunit (Guiroy et al. 1987). In the Guam PD-ALS complex, APC/ACA does not occur to any appreciable degree.

The N-terminal sequences of the NFT and APC showed considerable heterogeneity; the NFT more so than APC, and both more than ACA (Masters et al. 1985a, b; Pardridge et al. 1987). This suggested to us that in situ processing was occurring, and possibly that the degree of heterogeneity was a direct reflection of the age of the deposits.

The full length of the A4 molecule has now been sequenced and shown to consist of 42 or 43 residues (Kang et al. 1987) – one remarkable feature is the hydrophobic C-terminus (residues 30–42). As soon as the partial sequence of the A4 protein was determined, many groups around the world started performing gene cloning experiments to determine the structure of the precursor protein (the A4 product as such is small and unlikely to be derived as a primary translational product). At the same time, knowledge of the amino acid sequence permitted the construction of synthetic peptides which could then be used for studies of the biophysical nature of the A4 molecule, and also for raising antibodies to predetermined specificity.

The synthetic A4 material clearly showed that there are two regions in the molecule which are responsible for fibril formation. The synthetic fibrils closely match the native amyloid fibrils (Castaño et al. 1986; Kirschner et al. 1987). X-ray diffraction studies by Kirschner et al. (1986, 1987) and examination by infrared spectroscopy by our group showed that the basic packing of the subunit is as an antiparallel β-pleated sheet. This type of subunit orientation is similar to that found in other forms of amyloid fibrils (prealbumin, light chains of immunoglobulin, etc).

Monoclonal and polyclonal antisera raised against the A4 synthetic peptides and the native molecule are now proving to be most useful in the immunocytochemical demonstration of amyloid deposits in the AD-affected brain, in the DS-affected brain, and in the studies of amyloid deposits of aged normal animals such as the polar bear, the rhesus monkey, and the dog (Allsop et al. 1986; Bobin et al. 1987; Castaño et al. 1986; Davies et al. 1988; Masters et al. 1985b; Selkoe et al. 1987; Wong et al. 1985).

The A4 protein epitopes are not usually demonstrable on NFT, although some antisera to the N-terminal region of the A4 molecule do recognize a subpopulation of NFT (Masters et al. 1985b). Most antisera or histochemical reactions demonstrate a variety of adventitial molecules which may only be coating the surface of the PHF. These include neurofilament triplet protein (Anderton et al. 1982; Sternberger et al. 1985), ubiquitin (Mori et al. 1987), microtubule-associated protein 2 (Kosik et al. 1984), tau protein (Brion et al. 1985), ganglioside GQ1c (Emory et al. 1987) and sulfated glycosaminoglycans (Snow et al. 1987). Epitopes unique to NFT/PHF are also claimed (Ihara et al. 1983). In contrast, the A4 epitopes are readily demonstrable in situ in both APC and ACA, but even these structures also have adventitial molecules incorporated (Eikelenboom and Stam, 1982).

The gene (cDNA) coding for the A4 protein was partially sequenced by a number of workers (Goldgaber et al. 1987; Tanzi et al. 1987a; Robakis et al. 1987) and fully sequenced by Kang et al. (1987). The precursor protein (PreA4) has a predicted length of 695 residues, and has the structural domains typical of an integral membrane glycoprotein. PreA4 is not homologous with any other known protein. The A4 fragment is derived from a region of the molecule which encompasses part of the extracellular domain and part of the transmembrane region (thereby explaining its hydrophobic C-terminal region).

The A4 precursor gene is highly conserved, being present in all vertebrate species examined so far. The gene is expressed in most mammalian tissues (human and rodent) (Kang et al. 1987; Tanzi et al. 1987a; Goldgaber et al. 1987; Robakis et al. 1987), but expression in neurones is particularly evident from in situ hybridization studies (Bahmanyar et al. 1987; Goedert, 1987).

The A4 precursor gene is located in chromosome 21 (Kang et al. 1987; Tanzi et al. 1987a; Goldgaber et al. 1987; Robakis et al. 1987), at the junction of bands q21.3 and q22.1. This is very close, if not actually within, the region of chromosome 21 which must be duplicated for the phenotypic expression of DS. The gene is also present on the homologous mouse chromosome 16 (Lovett et al. 1987; Reeves et al. 1987).

St. George-Hyslop et al. (1987a) found linkage between the gene locus of FAD (young onset cases) and anonymous probes for the lng arm of chromosome 21. Using restriction fragment-length polymorphism analysis of FAD, it has now been shown by Van Broekhoven et al. (1987) and Tanzi et al. (1987b) that the FAD gene is distinct from the PreA4 gene. More than one gene for FAD may exist.

Initially it was thought that the PreA4 gene may be duplicated in AD (Delabar et al. 1987). We and others find no evidence for any form of duplication of the A4 precursor gene in sporadic and familial AD (Van Broeckhoven et al. 1987; Podlisny et al. 1987; St. George-Hyslop et al. 1987b; Tanzi et al. 1987c). The gene is duplicated in DS, and we now have biochemical evidence for the overexpression of this gene in DS but not in AD (Rumble et al. in preparation).

The normal function and the metabolism of the A4 precursor are now our primary targets for research. The PreA4 has a molecular mass of 90000–110000 daltons and is very labile. Its transmembrane orientation has been confirmed by in vitro translation experiments (Dyrks et al. 1988). The normal cellular location of the PreA4 is now being visualized using antisera to synthetic peptides corresponding to regions of the PreA4 molecule. In muscle, it is principally located at the perinuclear region of differentiated myofibers (Zimmermann et al. 1988).

We speculate that there are two distinct pathways involved in the pathogenesis of AD. The intracellular processing of PreA4 gives rise to A4 aggregates which form NFT; the extracellular processing of PreA4 gives rise to either APC or ACA. It is most likely that the main origin of the extracellular material is neuronal. In situ hybridization for mRNA shows a principal neuronal origin (Bahmanyar et al. 1987; Goedert 1987), and we are now awaiting the results of immunocytochemical studies.

Some investigators (Glenner and Wong 1984a, b; Selkoe et al. 1986) argue strongly for the hematogenous origin of the APC and ACA. We would argue equally strongly against this proposition on the following grounds:

a) The topographic distribution of APC/ACA does not correlate with any vascular territory or supply.
b) Deposition of ACA occurs in the outer walls of arterioles, less in capillaries, and least in venules.
c) There is often a demarcation of the deposition at the intima/media boundary in arterioles.
d) There is a preferential deposition in the Virchow-Robin space and in the overlying leptomeningeal arteries.
e) PreA4 has been localized to neurons by in situ hybridization and immuno-cytochemistry.
f) There is a relative lack of PreA4 in the liver and blood testing with Northern blots and radioimmunoassay.
g) An analogy can be made to the neuronal PrP, which polymerizes into APC/ACA in the unconventional virus diseases.

Is there one gene for AD? Given our present knowledge of the multiple steps likely to occur in the processing of PreA4, this now seems unlikely. Even if we can rule out overproduction of the A4 precursor, we are now faced with the prospect of multiple forms of the precursor, the mechanisms by which it is inserted and released from the cell membrane, and the processes which allow its degradative processing and the aggregation of the A4 subunit. A simple gene mutation or epimutation (Holliday 1987) may be involved in any step in this complicated pathway, but it is more likely that two or more errors combine to contribute to the formation of NFT/APC/ACA.

AD and Unconventional Virus Diseases

AD shares a number of clinical and pathological features with Creutzfeldt-Jakob disease (CJD), the human counterpart of scrapie in animals (Masters et al. 1981a); not least is the familial (autosomal dominant) inheritance of CJD and the occurrence of amyloid plaques and amyloid filaments in CJD (Masters et al. 1981b). The amyloid plaques occur as nonneuritic APC/ACA in all forms of the unconventional virus diseases, and are best seen in the Gerstmann-Straussler syndrome (GSS) (Masters et al. 1981b). The amyloid filaments, as in AD, occur in two forms: there is a distinctive scrapie-associated filament (SAF) (Merz et al. 1981) which bears some resemblance to the PHF, and there is a more typical amyloid filament with its presumed origin in the APC/ACA (Merz et al. 1983).

The principal protein component of the SAF is the PrP protein (Bolton et al. 1984; Prusiner et al. 1983) with a mass of 33000–35000 daltons. The gene for this protein is linked to genes which control the incubation period of scrapie (Carlson et al. 1986). The predicted structure of the PrP shows that it too is a membrane glycoprotein (Oesch et al. 1985) and in situ hybridization and immunocytochemical studies show that it is probably a neuronal membrane protein. Antisera to PrP and the direct biochemical analysis of the GSS APC show that the APC in these virus diseases is composed of PrP molecules. Since it appears that PrP plays an important role in the replication cycle of the infectious agent, it is logical to doubt whether PreA4 also participates in a similar process.

Many other etiological hypotheses for AD exist, some of which can be easily woven into the background of the studies now emerging on the A4 molecule and its role in amyloidogenesis. For example, if PreA4 requires membrane damage before it is released and becomes susceptible to amyloidogenic proteolytic cleavage, then theories and data which deal with lipid peroxidation, free radical attack, and oxidative stress should be sought (Martins et al. 1986). Do aluminosilicates play a role in the proteolytic degradation of PreA4 (Masters et al. 1985b; Candy et al. 1986)? These and other interesting questions (Holliday 1987) will form the basis for research into the cause of AD and its relationship to the normal aging of the brain.

References

Allsop D, Landon M, Kidd M, Lowe JS, Reynolds GP, Gardner A (1986) Monoclonal antibodies raised against a subsequence of senile plaque core protein react with plaque cores, plaque periphery and cerebrovascular amyloid in Alzheimer's disease. Neurosci Lett 68: 252–256

Anderton BH, Breinburg D, Downes MJ, Green PJ, Tomlinson BE, Ulrich J, Wood JN, Kahn J (1982) Monoclonal antibodies show that neurofibrillary tangles and neurofilaments share antigenic determinants. Nature 298: 84–86

Bahmanyar S, Higgins GA, Goldgaber D, Lewis DA, Morrison JH, Wilson MC, Shankar SK, Gajdusek DC (1987) Localization of amyloid β-protein messenger RNA in brains from Alzheimer's disease patients. Science 237: 77–80

Bobin SA, Currie JR, Merz PA, Miller DL, Styles J, Walker WA, Wen GY, Wisniewski HM (1987) The comparative immunoreactivities of brain amyloids in Alzheimer's disease and scrapie. Acta Neuropathol 74: 313–323

Bolton DC, McKinley MP, Prusiner SB (1984) Molecular characteristics of the major scrapie prion protein. Biochemistry 23: 5898–5906

Brion JP, van den Bosch de Aguilar P, Flament-Durand J (1985) Senile dementia of the Alzheimer type: morphological and immunocytochemical studies. In: Traber J, and Gispen WH (eds) Senile dementia of the Alzheimer type. Early diagnosis, neuropathology and animal models. Berlin, Springer, pp 164–174

Candy JM, Oakley AE, Klinowski J, Carpenter TA, Perry RH, Atack JR, Perry EK, Blessed G, Fairbairn A, Edwardson JA (1986) Aluminosilicates and senile plaque formation in Alzheimer's disease. Lancet 1: 354–357

Carlson GA, Kingsbury DT, Goodman PA, Coleman S, Marshall ST, DeArmond S, Westaway D, Prusiner SB (1986) Linkage of prion protein and scrapie incubation time genes. Cell 46: 503–511

Castaño EM, Ghiso J, Prelli F, Gorevic PD, Migheli A, Frangione B (1986) In vitro formation of amyloid fibrils from two synthetic peptides of different lengths homologous to Alzheimer's disease β-protein. Biochem Biophys Res Comm 141: 782–789

Davies L, Wolska B, Simms G, Kakulas BA, Masters CL, Hilbich C, Multhaup G, Beyreuther K (1988) Prevalence of the A4 amyloid protein of Alzheimer's disease in aged brains. Abstract submitted to the American Academy of Neurology

Delabar JM, Goldgaber D, Lamour Y, Nicole A, Huret JL, de Grouchy J, Brown P, Gajdusek DC, Sinet PM (1987) β-amyloid gene duplication in Alzheimer's disease and karyotypically normal Down syndrome. Science 235: 1390–1392

Dyrks T, Weidemann A, Multhaup G, Salbaum JM, Lemaire HG, Kang J, Müller-Hill B, Masters CL, Beyreuther K (1988) Identification, transmembrane orientation and biogenesis of the amyloid A4 precursor of Alzheimer's disease. Submitted for publication

Eikelenboom P, Stam FC (1982) Immunoglobulins and complement factors in senile plaques. Acta Neuropathol 57: 239–242

Emory CR, Ala TA, Frey WH (1987) Ganglioside monoclonal antibody (A2 B5) labels Alzheimer's neurofibrillary tangles. Neurology 37: 768–772

Glenner GG, Wong CW (1984a) Alzheimer's disease: initial report of the purification and characterization of a novel cerebrovascular amyloid protein. Biochem Biophys Res Comm 120: 885–890

Glenner GG, Wong CW (1984b) Alzheimer's disease and Down's syndrome: sharing of a unique cerebrovascular amyloid fibril protein. Biochem Biophys Res Comm 122: 1131–1135

Goedert M (1987) Neuronal localization of amyloid beta protein precursor mRNA in normal human brain and in Alzheimer's disease. EMBO J 6: 3627–3632

Goldgaber D, Lerman MI, McBride OW, Saffiotti U, Gajdusek DC (1987) Characterization and chromosomal localization of a cDNA encoding brain amyloid of Alzheimer's disease. Science 235: 877–880

Gorevic PD, Goñi F, Pons-Estel B, Alvarez F, Peress NS, Frangione B (1986) Isolation and partial characterization of neurofibrillary tangles and amyloid plaque core in Alzheimer's disease: immunohistological studies. J Neuropathol Exp Neurol 45: 647–664

Guiroy DC, Miyazaki M, Multhaup G, Fischer P, Garruto RM, Beyreuther K, Masters CL, Simms G, Gibbs CJ jr, Gajdusek DC (1987) Amyloid of neurofibrillary tangles of Guamanian parkinsonism-dementia and Alzheimer disease share identical amino acid sequence. Proc Natl Acad Sci USA 84: 2073–2077

Holliday R (1987) The interitance of epigenetic defects. Science 238: 163–170

Ihara Y, Abraham C, Selkoe DJ (1983) Antibodies to paired helical filaments in Alzheimer's disease do not recognize normal brain proteins. Nature 304: 727–730

Kang J, Lemaire H-G, Unterbeck A, Salbaum JM, Masters CL, Grzeschik K-H, Multhaup G, Beyreuther K, Muller-Hill B (1987) The precursor of Alzheimer's disease amyloid A4 protein resembles a cell-surface receptor. Nature 325: 733–736

Kirschner DA, Abraham C, Selkoe DJ (1986) X-ray diffraction from intraneuronal paired helical filaments and extraneuronal amyloid fibers in Alzheimer disease indicates cross-β conformation. Proc Natl Acad Sci USA 83: 503–507

Kirschner DA, Inouye H, Duffy LK, Sinclair A, Lind M, Selkoe DJ (1987) Synthetic peptide homologous to β-protein from Alzheimer disease forms amyloid-like fibrils in vitro. Proc Natl Acad Sci USA 84: 6953–6957

Kosik KS, Duffy LK, Dowling MM, Abraham C, McCluskey A, Selkoe DJ (1984) Microtubule-associated protein 2: monoclonal antibodies demonstrate the selective incorporation of certain epitopes into Alzheimer neurofibrillary tangles. Proc Natl Acad Sci USA 81: 7941–7945

Lovett M, Goldgaber D, Ashley P, Cox DR, Gajdusek DC, Epstein CJ (1987) The mouse homolog of the human amyloid β-protein (AD-AP) gene is located on the distal end of mouse chromosome 16: further extension of the homology between human chromosome 21 and mouse chromosome 16. Biochem Biophys Res Comm 144: 1069–1075

Martins RN, Harper CG, Stokes GB, Masters CL (1986) Increased cerebral glucose-6-phosphate dehydrogenase activity in Alzheimer's disease may reflect oxidative stress. J Neurochem 46: 1042–1045

Masters CL, Gajdusek DC, Gibbs CJ Jr (1981a) The familial occurrence of Creutzfeldt-Jakob and Alzheimer's disease. Brain 104: 535–558

Masters CL, Gajdusek DC, Gibbs CJ Jr (1981b) Creutzfeldt-Jakob disease virus isolation from the Gerstmann-Sträussler syndrome. With an analysis of the various forms of amyloid plaque deposition in the virus-induced spongiform encephalopathies. Brain 104: 559–587

Masters CL, Simms G, Weinman NA, Multhaup G, McDonald BL, Beyreuther K (1985a) Amyloid plaque core protein in Alzheimer disease and Down syndrome. Proc Natl Acad Sci USA 82: 4245–4249

Masters CL, Multhaup G, Simms G, Pottgiesser J, Martins RN, Beyreuther K (1985b) Neuronal origin of a cerebral amyloid: neurofibrillary tangles of Alzheimer's disease contain the same protein as the amyloid of plaque cores and blood vessels. EMBO J 4: 2757–2763

Merz PA, Somerville RA, Wisniewski HM, Iqbal K (1981) Abnormal fibrils from scrapie-infected brain. Acta Neuropathol 54: 63–74

Merz PA, Wisniewski HM, Somerville RA, Bobin SA, Masters CL, Iqbal K (1983) Ultrastructural morphology of amyloid fibrils from neuritic and amyloid plaques. Acta Neuropathol 60: 113–124

Mori H, Kondo J, Ihara Y (1987) Ubiquitin is a component of paired helical filaments in Alzheimer's disease. Science 235: 1641–1644

Oesch B, Westaway D, Wälchli M, McKinley MP, Kent SBH, Aebersold R, Barry RA, Tempst P, Teplow DB, Hood LE, Prusiner SB, Weissmann C (1985) A cellular gene encodes scrapie PrP 27–30 protein. Cell 40: 735–746

Pardridge WM, Winters HV, Yang J, Eisenberg J, Choi TB, Tourtellotte WW, Huebner V, Shively JE (1987) Amyloid angiopathy of Alzheimer's disease: amino acid composition and partial sequence of a 4,200-Dalton peptide isolated from cortical microvessels. J Neurochem 49: 1394–1401

Pearson RCA, Esiri MM, Hiorns RW, Wilcock GK, Powell TPS (1985) Anatomical correlates of the distribution of the pathological changes in neucortex in Alzheimer disease. Proc Natl Acad Sci USA 82: 4531–4535

Podlisny MB, Lee G, Selkoe DJ (1987) Gene dosage of the amyloid-β precursor protein in Alzheimer's disease. Science 238: 669–671

Prusiner SB, McKinley MP, Bowman KA, Bolton DC, Bendheim PE, Groth DF, Glenner GG (1983) Scrapie prions aggregate to form amyloid-like birefringent rods. Cell 35: 349–358

Reeves RH, Robakis NK, Oster-Granite ML, Wisniewski HM, Coyle JT, Gearhart JD (1987) Genetic linkage in the mouse of genes involved in Down syndrome and Alzheimer's disease in man. Molec Brain Res 2: 215–221

Robakis NK, Ramakrishna N, Wolfe G, Wisniewski HM (1987) Molecular cloning and characterization of a cDNA encoding the cerebrovascular and neuritic plaque amyloid peptides. Proc Natl Acad Sci USA 84: 4190–4194

Rogers J, Morrison JH (1985) Quantitative morphology and regional and laminar distributions of senile plaques in Alzheimer's disease. J Neurosci 5: 2801–2808

Selkoe DJ, Abraham CR, Podlisny MB, Duffy LK (1986) Isolation of low-molecular-weight proteins from amyloid plaque fibers in Alzheimer's disease. J Neurochem 46: 1820–1834

Selkoe DJ, Bell DS, Podlisny MB, Price DL, Cork LC (1987) Conservation of brain amyloid proteins in aged mammals and humans with Alzheimer's disease. Science 235: 873–877

Snow AD, Willmer JP, Kisilevsky R (1987) Sulfated glycosaminoglycans in Alzheimer's disease. Human Pathol 18: 506–510

Sternberger NH, Sternberger LA, Ulrich J (1985) Aberrant neurofilament phosphorylation in Alzheimer disease. Proc Natl Acad Sci USA 82: 4274–4276

St. George-Hyslop PH, Tanzi RE, Polinsky RJ, Haines JL, Nee L, Watkins PC, Myers RH, Feldman RG, Pollen D, Drachman D, Growdon J, Bruni A, Foncin JF, Salmon D, Frommelt P, Amaducci L, Sorbi S, Piacentini S, Stewart GD, Hobbs WJ, Conneally PM, Gusella JF (1987a) The genetic defect causing familial Alzheimer's disease maps on chromosome 21. Science 235: 885–890

St. George-Hyslop PH, Tanzi RE, Polinsky RJ, Neve RL, Pollen D, Drachman D, Growdon J, Cupples LA, Nee L, Myers RH, O'Sullivan D, Watkins PC, Amos JA, Deutsch CK, Bodfish JW, Kinsbourne M, Feldman RG, Bruni A, Amaducci L, Foncin JF, Gusella JF (1987b) Absence of duplication of chromosome 21 genes in familial and sporadic Alzheimer's disease. Science 238: 664–666

Tanzi RE, Gusella JF, Watkins PL, Bruns GAP, St. George-Hyslop P, van Keuren ML, Patterson D, Pagan S, Kurnit DM, Neve RL (1987a) Amyloid β-protein gene: cDNA, mRNA distribution, and genetic linkage near the Alzheimer locus. Science 235: 880–884

Tanzi RE, St. George-Hyslop PH, Haines JL, Polinsky RJ, Nee L, Foncin JF, Neve RL, McClatchey AI, Conneally PM, Gusella JF (1987b) The genetic defect in familial Alzheimer's disease is not tightly linked to the amyloid β-protein gene. Nature 329: 156–157

Tanzi RE, Bird ED, Latt SA, Neve RL (1987c) The amyloid β-protein gene is not duplicated in brains from patients with Alzheimer's disease. Science 238: 666–669

Van Broeckhoven C, Genthe AM, Vandenberghe A, Horsthemke B, Backhovens H, Raeymaekers P, Van Hul W, Wehnert A, Gheuens J, Cras P, Bruyland M, Martin JJ, Salbaum M, Multhaup G, Masters CL, Beyreuther K, Gurling HMD, Mullan MJ, Holland A, Barton A, Irving N, Williamson R, Richards SJ, Hardy JA (1987) Failure of familial Alzheimer's disease to segregate with the A4-amyloid gene in several European families. Nature 329: 153–155

Wong CW, Quaranta V, Glenner GG (1985) Neuritic plaques and cerebrovascular amyloid in Alzheimer disease are antigenically related. Proc Natl Acad Sci USA 82: 8729–8732

Zimmermann K, Herget T, Salbaum JM, Schubert W, Hilbich C, Cramer M, Masters CL, Multhaup G, Kang J, Lemaire H-G, Beyreuther K, Starzinski-Powitz A (1988) Localization of the putative precursor of Alzheimer's disease specific amyloid at nuclear envelopes of adult human muscle. EMBO J, in press

Genetics, Expression and Localization
of the Amyloid Precursor of Alzheimer's Disease

*K. Beyreuther, J. M. Salbaum, T. Dyrks, A. Genthe, A. Weidemann,
C. Hilbich, G. Multhaup, B. Horsthemke, P. Zabel,* and *C. L. Masters*

Summary

Alzheimer's disease is a neurodegenerative disorder of the cortex. The predominant
features of Alzheimer's disease are numerous amyloid depositions in the form of
plaques, vascular amyloid and neurofibrillary tangles. The A4 amyloid peptide is the
morphopoetic principle of the amyloid fibrils and the cleavage product of a larger
precursor protein. The gene for this A4 precursor encodes a primary translation
product of 695 amino acids (Masters et al., this volume).

The A4 precursor gene is located on chromosome 21 at the border between bands
q21 and q22.1 and much closer to the 21q22 Down's phenotype region than previously
reported (Tanzi et al. 1987).

We detected an intragenic restriction fragment length polymorphism with two
alleles, the allelic frequency being 0.65 versus 0.35 in caucasians. This BgL II restriction fragment length polymorphism for the A4 gene was used to track the inheritance
of the A4 gene through extensive pedigrees with early-onset familial Alzheimer's
disease and nuclear pedigrees with apparent late-onset Alzheimer's disease.

The resulting linkage data showed that the amyloid locus is only loosely linked to
the familial Alzheimer's disease locus and in two families a cross-over was observed
(Van Broeckhoven et al. 1987). This and the recent localization of the locus for
familial Alzheimer's disease (St. George Hyslop et al. 1987) indicate that a mutation
in the A4 amyloid precursor gene is not in all cases the primary defect causing familial
Alzheimer's disease.

Expression of the A4 gene is seen in brain, heart, muscle, kidney, adrenal gland,
lung, spleen, thymus, testes, and pancreas but not in liver. Using in situ hybridization
and immunocytochemistry, we discovered that A4 mRNA is ubiquitous and abundant
in gray matter; the protein appears as patches, predominantly on neuronal membranes, suggesting a role in cell contact for the A4 precursor protein (Shivers et al.
submitted).

References

St George-Hyslop PH, Tanzi RE, Polinski RJ, Haines JL, Nee L, Watkins PC, Myers RH, Feldman
RG, Pollen D, Drachman D, Growdon J, Bruni A, Foncin JF, Salmon D, Frommelt P, Amaducci
L, Sorbi S, Piacentini S, Stewart GD, Hobbs WJ, Conneally PM, Gusella JF (1987) The genetic
defect causing familial Alzheimer's disease maps on chromosome 21. Science 235: 885–890

Tanzi RE, Gusella JF, Watkins PC, Bruns GAP, St George-Hyslop P, Van Keuren ML, Patterson D, Pagan S, Kurnit DM, Neve RL (1987) Amyloid β protein gene: cDNA, mRNA distribution and genetic linkage near the Alzheimer locus. Science 235: 880–884
Van Broeckhoven C, Genthe AM, Vandenberghe A, Horsthemke B, Backhovens H, Raeymaekers P, Van Hul W, Wehnert A, Gheuens J, Cras P, Bruyland M, Martin JJ, Salbaum M, Multhaup G, Masters CL, Beyreuther K, Gurling HMD, Mullan MJ, Holland A, Barton A, Irving N, Williamson R, Richards SJ, Hardy JA (1987) Failure of familial Alzheimer's disease to segregate with the A4-amyloid gene in several European families. Nature 329: 153–155

Immunodiagnosis and Immunotherapy
of Patients with Alzheimer's Syndrome

H. H. Fudenberg, and *V. K. Singh*

Summary

We and others have shown unique structural and functional similarities of central nervous system (CNS) cells and peripheral blood immune cells. Hence, studies of various immune cells in peripheral blood make possible longitudinal studies of patients with CNS disorders, especially of the effects of therapy, without requiring serial brain biopsies. Using this approach in Alzheimer's disease (AD), we found aberrations of both cellular immunity and humoral immunity.

Depending upon the nature of the immune deficits and patients' responsiveness to appropriate immunomodulant therapy, we have thus far distinguished four subsets of AD patients: one subset with defect (membrane fluidity) of a specific T cell and who respond to pyrrolidone therapy; a second subset with serum antibodies to neuron-axon filament proteins – these patients improve clinically after therapy with dialyzable leucocyte extract (DLE); a third subset with antibodies to brain antigens (auto-immune) for whom therapy has not yet been developed; and a fourth subset with none of the abnormalities mentioned above, probably heterogeneous due to multiple biochemical deficiencies. We believe that different therapeutic modalities will be necessary for different subsets, much like the situation with other "diseases" such as anemia and diabetes. These results provide additional evidence that AD is a syndrome, not a single disease. Additionally, the clinical improvement demonstrated that the defective function in AD is not due to the relevant neuronal cells being dead, but because they are either atrophied or their function is suppressed.

Introduction

Alzheimer's Disease (AD) is a degenerative disorder of the central nervous system (CNS), characterized by impairment of memory, intellect, and cognitive functions in the early stages and by the loss of speech, ambulation, and bladder and rectal sphincter control in the later stages. The etiology and pathogenesis of the disease are unknown. However, current research suggests that the "disease" is in fact a syndrome, with different subsets caused by an infectious agent (a virus), dysfunction of the immune system, genetic predisposition, imbalance of trophic factors, and exposure to toxic substances (Fudenberg et al. 1984a; Wisniewski et al. 1985; Glenner 1985; Mann 1985).

We recently provided evidence that AD is a syndrome comprised of subsets with different etiologies, and that at least one subset is immunologic in origin (Fudenberg et al. 1984a; Singh et al. 1987). The rationale behind the study of the immune system in AD is derived from several lines of evidence:

1. The function of the cellular immune system declines with age, accompanied by an increased incidence of diseases (autoimmune) of aging (Weksler 1980; Vissinga et al. 1987).
2. There is an intriguing structural and functional relationship between the CNS and the immune system, especially demonstrated by the presence of neurotransmitter receptors on lymphocytes and the presence of lymphokine receptors on CNS cells (Singh and Fudenberg 1986a).
3. The predisposition of Down's syndrome patients to AD – Down's syndrome has been considered as a model of both accelerated aging and primary immunodeficiency (Walford et al. 1981; Burgio et al. 1983).
4. Immunologic mechanisms play an important role in other neurologic disorders (e.g., myasthenia gravis and multiple sclerosis), and patients with these diseases respond to immunotherapy (Dawkins and Garlepp 1985; Arnason 1985; Dabrowski et al. 1987).

The results of our immunologic studies, as reported herein, support our hypothesis that dysfunction of the immune system exists in AD patients, or at least in two subsets thereof. Because of functional and antigenic identities between the cells of the CNS and the immune system, we utilized tests of peripheral blood lymphocytes to measure the function of the corresponding CNS cells indirectly (Singh and Fudenberg 1986a). By using tests of blood immunocytes, we demonstrated that AD is not a single disease but rather a syndrome with differing etiologies, some with immunologic mechanisms; these respond to therapy with the appropriate immunomodulating agents.

Materials and Methods

Assessment of Cellular Immunity

The methods for measuring incorporation of [^{3}H]thymidine into lymphocyte DNA in response to stimulation by mitogens (phytohemagglutinin PHA; pokeweed mitogen, PWM; concanavalin A, Con A; anti-T_3 OKT$_3$), DNA synthesis of T cells stimulated by non-T cells (B cells and monocytes) in autologous mixed-lymphocyte reaction (AMLR), and the enumeration of orosomucoid (Om) positive T cells were essentially those described previously by us (Singh et al. 1987; Dirienzo et al. 1986).

Assessment of Humoral Immunity

Antibodies to brain tissue were detected by our method of indirect immunofluorescent histochemistry (Singh and Fudenberg 1986b). All sera were screened at 1:10 dilution using acetone-fixed frozen tissue sections of rat brain. The criterion of specific positive staining was as described previously (Singh and Fudenberg 1986b).

The analysis of serum IgG subclasses was performed with a radial immunodiffusion (RID) method (Singh and Fudenberg 1987) using RID plates from Serotec Ltd.

Serum antibodies to neuron-axon filament proteins (anti-NAFP) were detected using an immunoblot protein technique reported elsewhere (Galbraith et al. 1986). A positive reaction was observed against the high molecular weight protein band (200 kd) of rat spinal cord neurofilament preparations; a monoclonal antibody to it served as the positive control.

Subject Population

Immunologic profiles of 40 patients with AD were investigated. Controls included age-matched individuals and other disease controls. Patients included in the study had suffered from progressive symptoms for at least 2 years and showed cortical atrophy of the brain with no other abnormality on computed tomography, nonspecific EEG abnormalities, normal thyroid function, and normal vitamin B_{12} and folic acid levels. They had no history of cerebrovascular disease, no carotid artery stenoses, and were not taking any medication.

Therapy with Immunomodulating Agents

Our initial single-blind study of 23 AD patients with Piracetam, a nootropic pyrrolidone (Fudenberg et al. 1984b), showed that one subset of AD patients had a specific defect in one of the T cell subpopulations.

In the past 2–2½ years, we have studied 40 patients with AD in a double-blind crossover study with another nooleptic pyrrolidone Aniracetam (ANR) (Fig. 1), which is about 5 times more potent than Piracetam in in vitro assays using blood lymphocytes of patients with a deficiency in T cell function (H.H. Fudenberg, V.K. Singh, unpublished data). Patients were followed up for 2–5 years; each patient received either active medication (ANR; 0.5 g twice a day) or a placebo in the first arm of the study (3 months), followed by a 1-month "washout" period (without ANR or placebo). In the second crossover arm of the study (3 months), they were given the agent they had not received before, i.e., placebo if they had received ANR in the first arm or ANR if they had received placebo in the first arm. After completion of both arms of the study, patients who had responded clinically in either arm received another course of ANR without placebo for 6 months.

Results

In general, lymphocyte DNA synthesis in response to the mitogens listed in "Materials and Methods" was on the average lower than in normal age-matched controls, but there was considerable overlap (Fig. 1a). The data on AMLR and Om-positive T cells in AD patients were distributed in the same fashion as in the controls, but in a few cases the values were divisible into those higher and lower than in the controls (Fig. 1b, c).

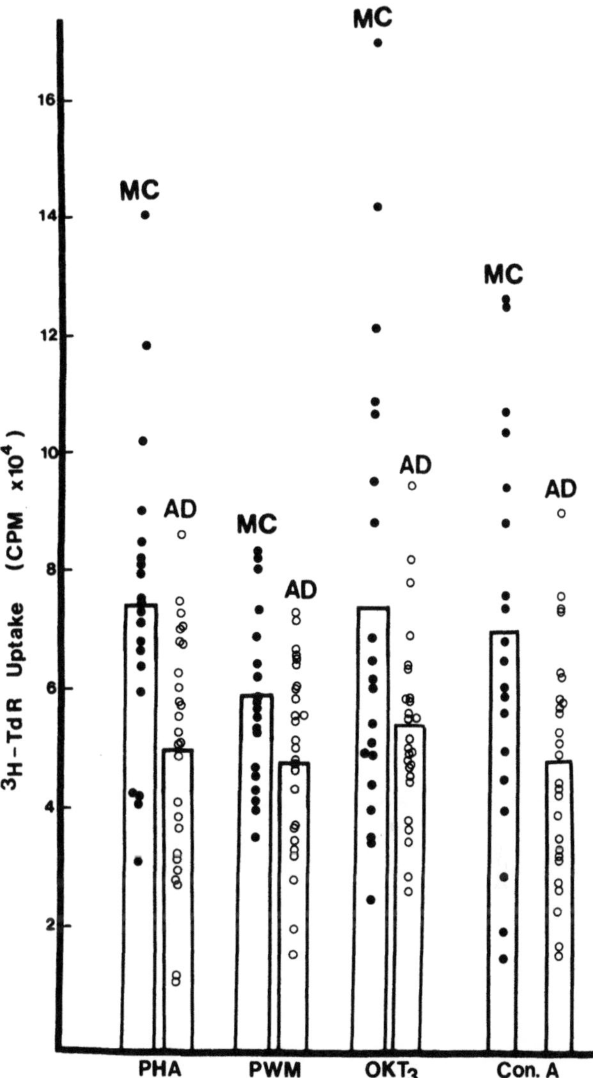

Fig. 1a–c. Results of lymphocyte DNA synthesis, AMLR- and orosomucoid-positive T cells. *Open circles* represent Alzheimer's disease *(AD)* and *solid circles* represent age-matched controls *(MC)*. **a** DNA synthesis, **b** AMLR, **c** Om⁺ T cells. *PHA,* phytohemagglutinin; *PWM,* pokeweed mitogen; *OKT₃,* anti-T₃; *ConA,* concanavalin A

With regards to humoral immunity, we found that about one-half of the patients tested had antibodies to brain antigens in their serum (Singh and Fudenberg 1986b). The nature of the brain antigen is not known but is currently under investigation. Analysis of serum IgG subclasses showed that the level of IgG_3, but not of IgG_1, IgG_2, or IgG_4, was elevated in nearly all patients who were positive for brain autoantibody; the sera with normal or low levels of IgG_3 uniformly lacked such autoantibody.

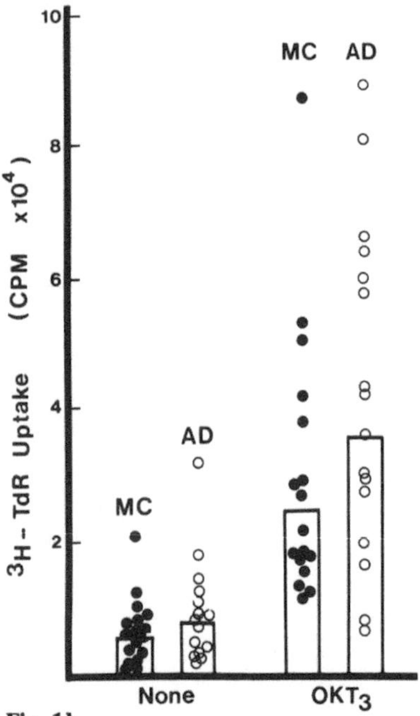

Fig. 1b

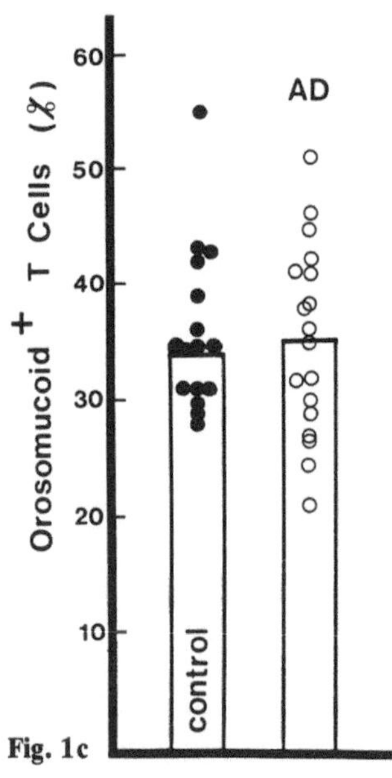

Fig. 1c

In other studies we found antibodies to NAFP in 13 (46%) of 28 sera tested by the immunoblot technique (Fig. 2). Positive results in this test are generally considered pathognomonic of past or present exposure to unconventional neurotropic viruses, whether or not disease results (Toh et al. 1985). Presumably, such viruses trigger cell-mediated immunity (CMI) and modify native constituents. We believe that the anti-NAFP is the result of an infection with an unconventional virus, and that it is not the cause of the disease. In some patients, 15 years elapsed between exposure to another AD patient and development of symptoms. Presumably, the viruses are kept latent by the host CMI mechanisms, and overt disease results only as CMI gradually decreases with aging.

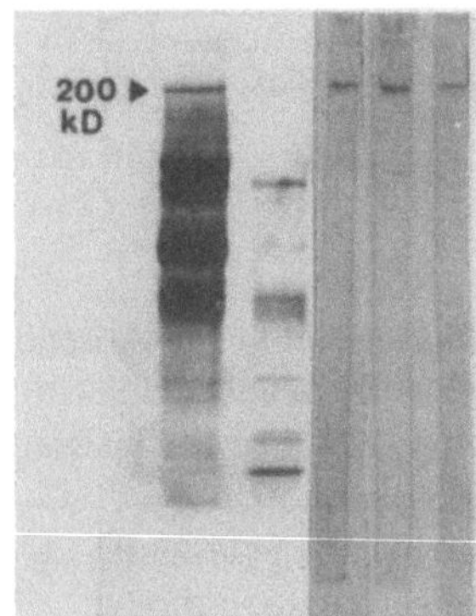

Fig. 2. Detection of antibodies to neuron-axon filament proteins (200 kd) in the sera of Alzheimer's disease patients and related controls

Eleven of the 40 patients responded to ANR therapy, as shown by improvement in both immunologic tests and clinical function in either the first or the second arm of the study. A few patients who had been clinical responders in a first study also participated in the second, and these patients again responded with improvements both in laboratory tests and clinically in one or other arm of the study. In contrast, among those patients who had failed to respond in the first study (Fudenberg et al. 1984b) and who also entered the second study, there was no clinical response in either arm of the second study. In the patients who improved clinically in one or other arm, improvement was seen from laboratory tests prior to clinical improvement becoming evident. Those who had improved in either arm of the study received, after completion of both arms, pyrrolidone without a placebo for 6 months. Thus, those who had received ANR in the second arm of the study received continuous therapy for 9 months, whereas those who had received ANR in the first arm were given only 6 months of uninterrupted therapy. The degree of improvement was not related to the duration or severity of the AD or to age at onset of illness, but rather was closely related to the duration of therapy (Fudenberg et al. 1984b; Singh and Fudenberg 1986c, d).

Additionally, we treated four AD patients with, and two without antibodies to NAFP with dialyzable leukocyte extract (DLE, containing transfer factor) obtained from immune cells of carefully selected blood donors. Each patient received DLE: 10 units (1 unit is the amount of DLE derived from 5×10^8 leukocytes) on the 1st day, 20 units on the 2nd day, 30 units on the 3rd day, and 40 units on the 4th day. The patients were then followed up for 30 days without being given additional DLE. Immunologic investigations before and after DLE therapy showed improvement of defective CMI in all six patients, but only those with antibodies to NAFP demonstrated a significant clinical response (Table 1). The two patients without such antibodies did not respond. These six patients were in stages IV to VI; three had recently lost the ability to ambulate and also had lost rectal and bladder sphincter control. By the 4th day of therapy, three of the patients were able to walk unaided, sphincter control improved, and there was dramatic improvement in cognitive function, as seen by spouse and friends. The clinical benefits lasted approximately 4 weeks (no therapy was given during this period), with gradual increase in disability thereafter. Readministration of DLE on the same schedule again resulted in marked clinical improvement similar in degree to that obtained after the first course of treatment.

Table 1. Results of various immune parameters and response to therapy with DLE

Patient code	Disease stage	Om^+T cells (%)	DNA synthesis[a] (+ PHA) (CPM)	Anti-NAFP[b]	Response to DLE therapy
D.M.	VI	34	35 135/ 38 483	+	++++
V.H.	V	36	31 309/ 49 148	+	+++
A.R.	VI	34	102 348/196 334	+	++
B.G.	V	30	23 011/ 63 212	−	+
S.H.	V	30	50 210/ 57 281	+	+
E.M.	IV	64	44 366/196 334	−	−

[a] Incorporation of [³H]thymidine into lymphocyte DNA (average of triplicate assays) for patient/control.
[b] Screened by the indirect immunofluorescent technique using frozen sections of rat spinal cord.

Discussion

Our results provide additional evidence for the concept that AD is not a single disease entity but a syndrome. At least one subset appears to be caused by an immune deficit which presumably disposes the patient to infection with unconventional viruses. The patients in this group responded to therapy with DLE, and the nature of clinical improvement indicates that, at least at stages IV to VI, the relevant cerebral cells in AD patients are not dead, but atrophied ("disuse atrophy"). This subset of AD patients, in addition to having the amyloid genes present on chromosome 21 (Van Broeckhoven et al. 1987; Tanzi et al. 1987), are presumably homozygous recessive for an unusual immune response gene (on chromosome 6) which precludes normal CMI response to unconventional viruses. Each spouse is presumably homozygous normal for the immune response gene to unconventional virus epitope(s) and the offspring are presumably heterozygous, which is why we prefer spouses to offspring as donors of blood cells for DLE. Since the gene coding for the superoxide dismutase enzyme is located between the genes coding for familial AD and cerebral amyloid on chromosome 21, we speculate that an imbalance in the activity of this enzyme (or one variant form of it), via tissue damage caused by a free oxygen radical, may be important in the abnormal formation of amyloid in the brain of patients with AD.

The "pyrrolidone subset" is of considerable interest in that 2-pyrrolidinone, an analogue of pyrrolidone, is present in high concentrations in CNS tissue and plasma. It is converted to succinimide by a series of enzymatic steps (Bandle et al. 1984). We hypothesize that one of a number (e.g., six or eight) of the enzymes in the pyrrolidinone pathway bypasses the block. This is similar to the situation in adrenocortical hyperplasia where a deficiency in any one of five enzymes produces identical clinical manifestations (White et al. 1987). The metabolic products of pyrrolidinones are necessary for the Krebs cycle metabolism of the cell. Normal energy metabolism appears necessary for normal membrane flexibility. The AD patients in this subset could conceivably have abnormal membrane fluidity (or flexibility), and pyrrolidones may bypass the enzymatic "block" and thereby restore normal membrane function. Our unpublished results showed that the addition of pyrrolidone to neuronal cells in cultures and blood lymphocytes produced about a 35% increase of neurotransmitter uptake.

Interestingly, abnormal membrane fluidity of platelets from AD patients was recently reported (Zubenko et al. 1987), providing some support for the hypothesis just mentioned. Our preliminary unpublished data on lymphocyte membrane studies of AD patients utilizing electron spin resonance (ESR) also support this concept.

A third subset of AD patients (autoimmune) is identified by the presence of circulating antibodies to brain tissue (Singh and Fudenberg 1986b) and an elevated level of serum IgG_3. The concentration of other subclasses was normal (Singh and Fudenberg 1987). It has been shown that the IgG_3 type of antibody is associated with the autoimmune phenomenon and/or infectious diseases (Beck 1981; Weetman and Cohen 1986; Rodgaard et al. 1987). The IgG_1 antibody is related to protein antigens whereas the IgG_2 and IgG_4 subclasses are directed against carbohydrate antigens (Siber et al. 1980; Hammarstrom and Smith 1986). Although the significance of our finding is unclear, it is tempting to speculate that such autoantibodies may be directed against intracellular or cell membrane constituents, e. g., glycoproteins, neurotransmitters (acetylcholine), or receptors for neurotransmitters. If so, this would explain the lack of efficacy of choline therapy in AD patients, since brain autoantibodies may bind to these neurons and interfere with their normal function. There is some evidence that antibrain antibodies are immunoreactive to cholinergic cells (Fillit et al. 1985). This subset may resemble the patients with autoimmune myasthenia gravis, in which autoantibodies bind to acetylcholine receptors and block the postsynaptic release of acetylcholine neurotransmitter at the neuromuscular junction. We are currently investigating the nature of the brain antigen in question, and will attempt to develop a rational therapy for this subset when the nature of the antigen provides a clue to its etiology.

Additional defects giving rise to other subtypes of AD patients can be envisioned, e. g., a genetic defect may exist in enzyme(s) necessary for oxidative metabolism in the brain cell equivalent (e. g., microglia) of one subset of blood monocytes, analogous to the enzymatic deficiency, e. g., of NADH oxidase, present in monocyte-derived cells in blood, liver, skin, etc., in chronic granulomatous disease (Ammann and Fudenberg 1976). Our other work (Chou et al. 1987) has shown the existence of four subsets of monocytes with the following characteristics:

1. The first has a high number of Fc receptors, high phagocytic function and no Ia antigen.
2. The second has no Fc receptors and no phagocytic function but is high in Ia antigen and is concerned with antigen presentation.
3. A third population produces immunologic inhibition via production of high levels of prostaglandin (PGE_2).
4. A fourth group produces high levels of a peptide-inhibitive interleukin-1 (IL-1) function.

Other monocyte defects in the subset of astrocytes, which are the brain equivalent of the antigen-presenting cells (Fontana et al. 1984), might result in underproduction of proteases predisposing to amyloid formation; overproduction of antiprotease would have the same effect. In this regard, it is noteworthy that α-1-antichymotrypsin, a protease inhibitor which reacts with many proteases in addition to chymotrypsin, was recently found in the cerebral amyloid (see Selkoe this volume). Presumably, nonimmune parameters also serve as etiologic factors, e. g., biochemical and/or functional abnormality of neurotransmitters (acetylcholine) and/or neuropeptides (somatostatin, corticotropin releasing factor).

Based upon the results presented above, we conclude that AD is not a single disease, but rather a syndrome involving multiple etiological factors. This view is supported by our observations of the existence of aberrations of both cellular and humoral immunity, in particular, of autoimmunity. Additionally, we have discerned subcategories of immunologically defined subsets of AD patients. Appropriate therapy in each patient depends upon the nature of the deficit and predicts the responsiveness. New therapies will necessitate knowledge of the etiology in each patient. Therapies for each subset will differ, just as is the case with various forms of anemia, diabetes, and other diseases. Finally, we stress that regaining of function with therapy implies that CNS cells are not dead but merely atrophied or functionally suppressed.

Acknowledgment. This work was supported by the Immunohematology Research Foundation. The authors would like to thank Emily Paulling and Joan Emerick for their excellent technical assistance.

References

Ammann AJ, Fudenberg HH (1976) Immunodeficiency diseases. In: Fudenberg HH, Stites DP, Caldwell JL, Wells JV (eds) Basic and clinical immunology. Lange Medical, Los Altos, CA, pp 391–421

Arnason BG (1985) Multiple sclerosis, allied central nervous system diseases, and immune-mediated neuropathies. In: Rose NR, Mackay IR (eds) The autoimmune diseases. Academic, New York, pp 399–427

Bandle EF, Wendt G, Ranalder UB, Trautmann KH (1984) 2-Pyrrolidinone and succinimide endogenously present in several mammalian species. Life Sci 35: 2205–2212

Beck OE (1981) Distribution of virus antibody activity among human IgG subclasses. Clin Exp Immunol 43: 626–632

Burgio GR, Ugazio A, Nespoli L, Maccario R (1983) Down's syndrome: a model of immunodeficiency. Birth Defects 19: 325–327

Chou YK, Stanley W, Virella G, Kilpatrick JM, Fudenberg HH (1987) Generation of phenotypically distinct macrophage-hepatoma hybrid clones. Immunobiology, in press

Dabrowski MP, Bernstein BK, Stasiak A, Gajkowski K, Korniluk S (1987) Immunologic and clinical evaluation of multiple sclerosis patients treated with corticosteroids and/or calf thymic hormones. Ann NY Acad Sci 496: 697–706

Dawkins RL, Garlepp MJ (1985) Autoimmune diseases of muscle: myasthenia gravis and myositis. In: Rose NR, Mackay IR (eds) The autoimmune diseases. Academic, New York, pp 591–615

Dirienzo W, Stefanini GF, Singh VK, Paulling EE, Canonica GW, Fudenberg HH (1986) Does normal lymphocyte DNA synthesis in response to PHA exclude cell-mediated immunodepression? Clin Immunol Immunopathol 41: 227–235

Fillit H, Luine VN, Reisberg B, Amador R, McEwen B, Zabriskie JB (1985) Studies of the specificity of antibrain antibodies in Alzheimer's disease. Neurol Neurobiol 18: 307–318

Fontana A, Fierz W, Wekerle H (1984) Astrocytes present myelin basic protein to encephalitogenic T-cell lines. Nature 307: 273–276

Fudenberg HH, Whitten HD, Arnaud P, Khansari N (1984a) Is Alzheimer's disease an immunological disorder? Observations and speculations. Clin Immunol Immunopathol 32: 127–131

Fudenberg HH, Whitten HD, Arnaud P, Khansari N, Tsang KY, Hames CG (1984b) Immune diagnosis of a subset of Alzheimer's disease with preliminary implications for immunotherapy. Biomed Pharmacother 38: 290–297

Galbraith GMP, Emerson D, Fudenberg HH, Gibbs CJ, Gajdusek DC (1986) Antibodies to neurofilament protein in retinitis pigmentosa. J Clin Invest 78: 865–869

Glenner GG (1985) On causative theories in Alzheimer's disease. Hum Pathol 16: 433–435

Hammarstrom L, Smith CIE (1986) Immunoglobulin isotype diversity and its functional significance. In: French MAH (ed) Immunoglobulins in health and disease. MTP, London, pp 31–53

Mann DMA (1985) The neuropathology of Alzheimer's disease: a review with pathogenic, etiological and therapeutic considerations. Mech Ageing Dev 31: 213–255

Rodgaard A, Nielsen FC, Djurup R, Somnier F, Gammeltoft S (1987) Acetylcholine receptor antibody in myasthenia gravis: predominance of IgG subclasses 1 and 3. Clin Exp Immunol 67: 82–88

Siber G, Schur PH, Aisenberg AC, Weitzman SA, Schiffman G (1980) Correlation between serum IgG-2 concentrations and the antibody response to bacterial polysaccharide antigens. N Engl J Med 303: 178–182

Singh VK, Fudenberg HH (1986a) Can blood immunocytes be used to study neuropsychiatric disorders? J Clin Psychiatry 47: 592–595

Singh VK, Fudenberg HH (1986b) Detection of brain autoantibodies in the serum of patients with Alzheimer's disease but not Down's syndrome. Immunol Lett 12: 277–280

Singh VK, Fudenberg HH (1986c) Immunologic approach to etiology and therapy of neuropsychiatric disorders. In: Bignami A, Bolis L, Gadjusek DC (eds) Molecular mechanisms for pathogenesis of central nervous system disorders, F.E.S.N. Discussion in Neurosciences, vol 3, pp 120–124

Singh VK, Fudenberg HH (1986d) Immunopharmacological approach to the study of chronic brain disorders. Prog Drug Res 30: 345–363

Singh VK, Fudenberg HH (1987) Increase of immunoglobulin G_3 subclass is related to brain autoantibody in Alzheimer's disease but not in Down's syndrome. J Clin Immunol, in press

Singh VK, Fudenberg HH, Brown FR III (1987) Immunologic dysfunction: simultaneous study of Alzheimer's and older Down's patients. Mech Ageing Dev 37: 257–264

Tanzi RE, St. George-Hyslop PH, Haines JL, Polinsky RJ, Nee L, Foncin JF, Neve RL, McClatchey AI, Conneally PM, Gusella JF (1987) The genetic defect in familial Alzheimer's disease is not tightly linked to the amyloid beta-protein gene. Nature 329: 156–157

Toh BH, Gibbs CJ, Gajdusek DC, Goudsmit J, Dahl D (1985) The 200- and 150-kDa neurofilament proteins react with IgG autoantibodies from patients with kuru, Creutzfeldt-Jacob disease, and other neurological diseases. Proc Natl Acad Sci USA 82: 3485–3489

Van Broeckhoven C, Genthe AM, Vandenberghe A, Horsthemke B, Backhovens H, Raeymaekers P, Van Hul W, Wehnert A, Gheuens J, Cras P, Bruyland M, Martin JJ, Salbaum M, Multhaup G, Masters CL, Beyreuther K, Gurling HMD, Mullan MJ, Holland A, Barton A, Irving N, Williamson R, Richards SJ, Hardy JA (1987) Failure of familial Alzheimer's disease to segregate with the A4-amyloid gene in several European families. Nature 329: 153–155

Vissinga CS, Dirven CJAM, Dirven FA, Steinmeyer VA, Benner R, Boersma WJA (1987) Deterioration of cellular immunity during aging. The relationship between age-dependent impairment of delayed-type hypersensitivity reactivity, interleukin-2 production capacity, and frequency of $Thy1^+$, $Lyt-2^-$ cells in C57BL/Ka and CBA/Rij mice. Cell Immunol 108: 323–334

Walford RL, Gossett TC, Naeim F, Tam CF, Van Lancker JL, Bennett EV, Chia D, Sparkes RS, Fahey JL, Spina C, Gatti RA, Medici MA, Grossman H, Hibrawi H, Motola M (1981) Immunological and biochemical studies of Down's syndrome as a model of accelerated aging. In: Segre D, Smith L (eds) Immunological aspects of aging. Dekker, New York, pp 479–532

Weetman AP, Cohen S (1986) The IgG subclass distribution of thyroid autoantibodies. Immunol Lett 13: 335–341

Weksler ME (1980) The immune system and the aging process in man. Proc Soc Exp Biol Med 165: 200–203

White PC, New MI, Dupont B (1987) Congenital adrenal hyperplasia. N Engl J Med 316: 1519–1524

Wisniewski HM, Merz GS, Carp RI (1985) Current hypothesis of the etiology and pathogenesis of senile dementia of the Alzheimer's type. Interdisc Top Gerontol 19: 45–53

Zubenko GS, Cohen BM, Reynolds CF, Boller F, Malinakova I, Keefe N (1987) Platelet membrane fluidity in Alzheimer's disease and major depression. Am J Psychiatry 144: 860–868

Subject Index